# NUTRITION AND DIET

## Characteristics of health And fitness

## By

## Emmanuel Noble

# TABLE OF CONTENTS

# INTRODUCTION OF NUTRITION AND DIET..

*"**Nutrition** is the cornerstone of our existence, influencing our health, energy levels, and overall well-being. It's the science that examines the relationship between the food we eat and the impact it has on our bodies. Understanding nutrition is crucial because it empowers us to make informed choices about what we eat, ensuring that we provide our bodies with the necessary nutrients to thrive. In this book, we'll embark on a journey through the fascinating world of nutrition, exploring the role of essential nutrients, the effects of various diets, and the profound connection between what we eat and how we feel. Together, we'll unravel the secrets of nutrition and discover how to make healthier dietary choices for a better, more vibrant life."*

# CHAPTER 1

The "Introduction to Nutrition" chapter is an essential starting point for your book on nutrition and diet. This chapter provides readers with a foundation for understanding the core concepts and importance of nutrition. Here's a more detailed explanation of what this chapter may include:

1. **Definition of Nutrition:** *Begin by defining what nutrition is. Explain that it is the science that deals with the relationship between living organisms and the food they consume. Nutrition encompasses the study of nutrients, their sources, their functions in the body, and their effects on health.*

2. **Historical Perspective:** *Briefly touch upon the historical context of nutrition. Describe how our understanding of nutrition has evolved over time, from ancient dietary practices to modern scientific discoveries.*

3. ***Why Nutrition Matters:** Emphasize the critical role nutrition plays in maintaining overall health and well-being. Discuss how proper nutrition can prevent chronic diseases, support growth and development, and improve the quality of life.*

4. ***The Components of Food:** Introduce the main components of food, which are macronutrients (carbohydrates, proteins, fats) and micronutrients (vitamins and minerals). Explain how these nutrients are essential for various bodily functions.*

5. ***Energy Balance:** Discuss the concept of energy balance, highlighting the importance of matching the energy consumed through food with the energy expended through physical activity. Explain how this balance affects body weight.*

6. ***Nutritional Guidelines:** Mention the existence of dietary guidelines and recommendations set by health authorities or organizations in various countries. These guidelines can serve as a reference point for making healthy food choices.*

7. ***The Connection to Disease:** Introduce the idea that nutrition is closely linked to the prevention and management of diseases, including obesity, diabetes, heart disease, and more.*

8. ***Personalized Nutrition:** Touch on the emerging field of personalized nutrition, where individuals consider*

*their unique genetic makeup and lifestyle when making dietary choices.*

# CHAPTER 2

## History of Nutrition

*The history of nutrition is a fascinating journey that highlights the evolving understanding of the relationship between food and human health.*

1. **Ancient Dietary Practices:** *Begin with a look at how early civilizations, such as the Egyptians, Greeks, and Romans, approached food and nutrition. Explain their beliefs and practices related to diet.*

2. **Hippocrates and the Humoral Theory**: *Discuss the significant contributions of Hippocrates, often regarded as the father of medicine. His humoral theory, which connected health with the balance of bodily fluids, played a pivotal role in ancient nutrition concepts.*

3. **Vitamins and Early Discoveries:** *Move forward in time to the 18th and 19th centuries when early scientists like James Lind (known for his work on scurvy) began to understand the importance of specific nutrients.*

4. **The Birth of Modern Nutrition Science:** *Explore the 20th century when the field of nutrition as we know it today began to take shape. Mention the pioneering work of scientists like Casimir Funk, who coined the term*

"vitamin," and Elmer McCollum and Marguerite Davis, who discovered vitamins A and B.

5. **World Wars and Nutrition:** Highlight the role of nutrition in wartime, as both World War I and World War II brought attention to the importance of feeding soldiers and the impact of malnutrition.

6. **The Discovery of Macronutrients** Discuss the identification and Understanding of macronutrients, including carbohydrates, proteins, and fats, and how they became central to dietary recommendations.

7. **Nutrition Guidelines:** Explain how governments and health organizations began to establish dietary guidelines, such as the food pyramid, to promote healthier eating habits.

8. **Nutritional Milestones:** Touch upon significant milestones in nutrition science, including the discovery of essential amino acids and fatty acids, and the development of tools to measure nutritional content.

9. **The Role of Nutrigenomics:** Briefly mention the relatively recent field of nutrigenomics, which explores how our genes influence our response to nutrients and dietary choices.

10. **Current Trends and Challenges:** Conclude by noting the current trends and challenges in nutrition, such as the rise of processed foods, obesity, and the

*ongoing quest to understand the complex interplay between diet and health.*

# CHAPTER 3.

## **The Science of Nutrition:** Understanding the Art of Eating for Health.

*Nutrition is the science that explores how the body processes and uses the food we consume to maintain and improve health. It involves the study of nutrients, their functions, and how different dietary choices impact our well-being. Here's a comprehensive explanation of the science of nutrition:*

*1. **Nutrients:** The Building Blocks of Nutrition*
*Nutrients are the essential components of food that the body requires for growth, energy, and overall health. They are divided into two main categories:*
   ***Macronutrients:** These include carbohydrates, proteins, and fats, which provide energy and are needed in large quantities.*
   ***Micronutrients:** These include vitamins and minerals, which are required in smaller amounts but are crucial for various bodily functions.*

*2. **Digestion and Absorption:** Unlocking Nutrient Potential*
   *The process of nutrition begins with digestion, where food is broken down into its constituent nutrients. These*

nutrients are then absorbed by the body and transported to cells for energy and growth.

**3. Energy Balance and Metabolism:** Fueling the Body
Nutrition is closely tied to energy balance, which is the equilibrium between the calories consumed and the calories expended. The body uses this energy for basic functions like breathing and metabolism, as well as physical activity.
Metabolism is the set of chemical processes that convert food into energy and support the body's functions. Understanding how metabolism works is central to the science of nutrition.

**4. Essential Nutrients:** The Body's Nutritional Needs
Essential nutrients are those the body cannot produce in sufficient quantities and must be obtained through diet. They include carbohydrates, proteins, fats, vitamins, and minerals. A well-balanced diet ensures that these essential nutrients are provided.

**5. Dietary Guidelines:** Science-Based Recommendations
Nutrition science informs dietary guidelines issued by health authorities to promote a healthy diet. These guidelines help individuals make informed food choices that support overall health and prevent nutritional deficiencies and chronic diseases.

**6. Special Diets:** Catering to Unique Needs

*Nutrition science addresses the nutritional needs of individuals with specific requirements, such as athletes, pregnant women, children, and those with medical conditions like diabetes or celiac disease.*

*Specialized diets like vegetarian, vegan, ketogenic, and paleo diets also fall under the purview of nutrition science.*

**7. Nutritional Myths and Facts:** *Navigating Information*
*Nutrition is a field marked by a wealth of information, some of which is misleading. The science of nutrition helps distinguish between nutritional myths and evidence-based facts, enabling individuals to make informed choices.*

**8. Food and Health: Prevention and Treatment**
*Nutrition science plays a pivotal role in preventing and managing chronic diseases like heart disease, obesity, and diabetes. Specific diets and nutritional strategies can be prescribed to improve health and well-being.*

**9. Future of Nutrition: Evolving Trends**
*The field of nutrition is constantly evolving. Trends and innovations in personalized nutrition, functional foods, sustainability, and food transparency are shaping the future of this science.*

*In conclusion, the science of nutrition is integral to our understanding of how food impacts our bodies and our health. It guides us in making informed dietary choices that support well-being and prevent disease, emphasizing the importance of a balanced diet that provides essential nutrients, promotes energy balance, and fuels our metabolism.*

# CHAPTER 4

In a chapter on **"Essential Nutrients: Carbohydrates,"** you can explore the role of carbohydrates in our diet and their significance for overall health. Here's a breakdown of what you can include in this chapter:

*1. Introduction to Carbohydrates* *Begin by defining carbohydrates as one of the three primary macronutrients, alongside proteins and fats. Explain that they are the body's main source of energy.*

*2. Carbohydrate Classification:*
*Describe the two main categories of carbohydrates: simple carbohydrates (sugars) and complex carbohydrates (starches and fiber).*

*3. Sources of Carbohydrates:* *List common food sources of carbohydrates, including grains, fruits, vegetables, legumes, and dairy products.*

*4. Carbohydrates and Energy:* *Explain how carbohydrates are efficiently converted into glucose, which is used by the body as its primary energy source.*

**5. Glucose Metabolism:** *Detail the process of glucose metabolism, including glycolysis and the role of insulin in regulating blood sugar levels.*

**6. Dietary Fiber:** *Discuss the importance of dietary fiber in maintaining digestive health, preventing constipation, and reducing the risk of certain diseases.*

**7. Glycemic Index:** *Introduce the concept of the glycemic index (GI) and how it measures the impact of carbohydrates on blood sugar levels. Explain how low-GI foods are often considered healthier choices.*

**8. Carbohydrates and Brain Function:** *Describe the role of carbohydrates in supporting brain function and mental clarity, emphasizing the need for adequate glucose supply.*

**9. Carbohydrates in Sports Nutrition:** *Discuss the significance of carbohydrates for athletes and active individuals, as they provide quick energy for physical activities.*

**10. Carbohydrates and Weight Management:** *Explain the relationship between carbohydrate consumption, satiety, and weight management. Address common misconceptions about carbohydrates and weight gain.*

**11. Carbohydrates and Health:** *Explore the impact of carbohydrates on overall health, including their role in reducing the risk of chronic diseases like heart disease and type 2 diabetes when consumed in a balanced diet.*

**12. Recommendations and Daily Intake:** *Provide general guidelines for the recommended daily intake of carbohydrates, and mention how it can vary based on an individual's age, gender, and activity level.*

**13. Low-Carbohydrate Diets:** *Discuss low-carb diets like the ketogenic diet and their potential benefits and drawbacks. Emphasize the importance of balance in dietary choices.*

**14. Carbohydrate Myths and Facts.** *Address common myths and misconceptions about carbohydrates, such as the idea that all carbs are bad or that they should be completely eliminated from the diet.*

**15. Practical Tips for Carbohydrate Consumption:** *Offer practical tips for readers on how to make healthier carbohydrate choices, including choosing whole grains, fruits, and vegetables over sugary and processed foods.*

*This chapter should provide readers with a comprehensive understanding of carbohydrates, their role in nutrition, and how to make informed choices about carbohydrate consumption to support overall health and well-being.*

# CHAPTER 5

## Protein: The Building Blocks of Life

*Proteins are one of the essential nutrients that play a fundamental role in the structure and function of the human body. They are often referred to as the "building blocks of life" for good reason. Here's a comprehensive explanation of proteins and their significance:*

### 1. What Are Proteins?
*Proteins are large, complex molecules composed of amino acids. They are found in various foods, with the richest sources being meat, poultry, fish, dairy products, eggs, legumes, and nuts.*

### 2. Functions of Proteins:
*Proteins serve a wide range of essential functions in the body, including:*

*__Structural Role:__ Proteins are the building blocks of cells, tissues, and organs. They provide the structural framework for muscles, bones, skin, hair, and enzymes.*

*__Enzymes:__ Many biological reactions in the body are facilitated by enzymes, which are specialized proteins that act as catalysts.*

*__Hormones:__ Some hormones, like insulin and growth hormone, are proteins that regulate various physiological processes.*

**Immune Function:** *Antibodies are proteins that help the immune system defend the body against pathogens.*

**Transport:** *Hemoglobin is a protein that transports oxygen in the blood. Other proteins transport molecules across cell membranes.*

**Energy Production:** *While carbohydrates are the primary energy source, proteins can be broken down for energy when carbohydrates are insufficient.*

### 3. Amino Acids:

*Amino acids are the building blocks of proteins. There are 20 different amino acids, and they can be combined in various sequences to form countless proteins.*

*Of these amino acids, nine are aaàconsidered essential because the body cannot produce them, and they must be obtained through the diet.*

### 4. Protein Quality:

*The quality of a protein source is determined by its amino acid profile. Animal-based proteins are typically considered high-quality because they contain all essential amino acids in sufficient amounts.*

*Plant-based proteins may lack certain amino acids, but a balanced diet with a variety of plant foods can provide adequate protein and amino acids.*

### 5. Recommended Protein Intake:

*The recommended daily protein intake varies based on factors such as age, gender, activity level, and health status. In general, protein should make up about 10-35% of daily caloric intake.*

### 6. Health Considerations:

Protein deficiency can lead to muscle wasting, weakness, and impaired growth and development, especially in children.

Excessive protein intake may strain the kidneys and be associated with some health risks, such as kidney stones and bone health issues.

### 7. Dietary Sources:

Excellent sources of protein include lean meats, poultry, fish, dairy products, eggs, legumes (beans, lentils), nuts, and seeds.

Vegetarians and vegans can obtain protein from plant sources like tofu, tempeh, legumes, and whole grains.

In conclusion, proteins are vital nutrients that play a multifaceted role in maintaining and promoting health. Including a variety of protein sources in your diet ensures that you obtain the necessary amino acids and support the body's structure, function, and overall well-being.

# CHAPTER 6.

## **Essential Nutrients:** Fats - Fueling and Protecting Your Body

*Fats are a class of essential nutrients that are vital for various physiological functions in the body. While they have been associated with negative connotations in the past, fats are crucial for overall health. Here's a comprehensive explanation of fats and their significance:*

### *1. What Are Fats?*

*Fats, also known as lipids, are organic molecules made up of carbon, hydrogen, and oxygen atoms. They come in various forms, including saturated fats, unsaturated fats, and trans fats.*

### *2. Functions of Fats:*

*Fats play several essential roles in the body, including:*

***Energy Storage:** Fats are the most concentrated source of energy, providing long-term reserves of fuel.*

**Cell Membranes:** *Fats are integral components of cell membranes, helping to maintain their structure and function.*

**Absorption of Fat-Soluble Vitamins:** *Fats facilitate the absorption of fat-soluble vitamins (A, D, E, and K).*

**Protection of Organs:** *Fat acts as a protective cushion around vital organs.*

**Insulation:** *Subcutaneous fat insulates the body and helps maintain temperature.*

**Brain Health:** *Omega-3 fatty acids are critical for brain development and function.*

### *3. Types of Fats:*

*Fats can be categorized into three main types:*

**Saturated Fats:** *These fats are typically solid at room temperature and are found in animal products, tropical oils, and some processed foods. A high intake of saturated fats has been linked to an increased risk of heart disease.*

**Unsaturated Fats:** *Unsaturated fats can be further divided into monounsaturated and polyunsaturated fats. They are usually liquid at room temperature and are considered heart-healthy. Sources include olive oil, avocados, and fatty fish.*

**Trans Fats:** *Trans fats are artificially created through a process called hydrogenation and are found in some processed and fried foods. They are associated with an increased risk of heart disease and are being phased out in many places.*

### *4. Essential Fatty Acids:*

*The body cannot produce certain fatty acids, such as omega-3 and omega-6 fatty acids, on its own. These are referred to as essential fatty acids and must be obtained through the diet. They are critical for brain health, inflammation regulation, and overall well-being.*

### 5. Balanced Fat Intake:
*A balanced diet includes a variety of fats, with an emphasis on unsaturated fats, including omega-3 fatty acids found in fatty fish (e.g., salmon, mackerel) and walnuts. Reducing the consumption of saturated and trans fats is essential for heart health.*

### 6. Recommended Fat Intake:
*Fat should make up about 20-35% of daily caloric intake, with the majority coming from healthy sources like nuts, seeds, and plant-based oils.*

### 7. Health Considerations:
*Fats are calorie-dense, so portion control is essential to maintain a healthy weight.*
*Monounsaturated and polyunsaturated fats can help lower the risk of heart disease when they replace saturated and trans fats in the diet.*

### 8. Dietary Sources:
*Sources of healthy fats include olive oil, avocados, nuts, seeds, fatty fish, and plant-based oils like canola and flaxseed oil.*

*In conclusion, fats are essential nutrients that play multiple roles in maintaining and promoting health. Including a variety of healthy fats in your diet ensures that you receive the benefits of essential fatty acids and support the body's energy, structure, and overall well-being.*

# CHAPTER 7

## Water-Soluble Vitamins: Essential Nutrients Dissolved in Hydration

*Water-soluble vitamins are a group of essential nutrients that are soluble in water and must be obtained regularly through the diet. They include the B-complex vitamins (B1, B2, B3, B5, B6, B7, B9, B12) and vitamin C. Here's a comprehensive explanation of water-soluble vitamins and their significance:*

### 1. Types of Water-Soluble Vitamins:
*The B-complex vitamins include thiamine (B1), riboflavin (B2), niacin (B3), pantothenic acid (B5), pyridoxine (B6), biotin (B7), folate (B9), and cobalamin (B12).*

*Vitamin C, also known as ascorbic acid, is another water-soluble vitamin.*

### 2. Functions of Water-Soluble Vitamins:
*Water-soluble vitamins play various essential roles in the body:*

***Energy Metabolism:*** *Many B vitamins are involved in converting the food we eat into energy. They act as coenzymes in metabolic reactions.*

***Cell Growth and Development:***

*Folate (B9) is essential for cell division and is crucial during pregnancy.*

**Immune Function:** *Vitamin C is known for its role in supporting the immune system and acting as an antioxidant.*

**Nervous System Health:** *Several B vitamins are essential for proper nerve function and the synthesis of neurotransmitters.*

### 3. Solubility and Absorption:

*Water-soluble vitamins are easily dissolved in water and absorbed directly into the bloodstream through the digestive tract.*

*Unlike fat-soluble vitamins (A, D, E, and K), water-soluble vitamins are not stored in the body for long periods. Excess amounts are excreted through urine, making regular intake important.*

### 4. Dietary Sources:

*Water-soluble vitamins are found in a wide range of foods, including:*

*Thiamine (B1): Whole grains, pork, and legumes.*

*Riboflavin (B2): Dairy products, lean meats, and green leafy vegetables.*

*Niacin (B3): Meat, poultry, fish, and enriched cereals.*

*Pantothenic Acid (B5): Found in virtually all foods.*

*Pyridoxine (B6): Meat, fish, nuts, and fortified cereals.*

*Biotin (B7): Liver, egg yolk, and nuts.*

*Folate (B9): Leafy greens, legumes, and fortified cereals.*

*Cobalamin (B12): Found primarily in animal products.*
*Vitamin C: Citrus fruits, strawberries, bell peppers, and broccoli.*

### 5. Recommended Intake:
*Adequate intake of water-soluble vitamins varies based on age, gender, and specific health needs. They are usually expressed as recommended daily allowances (RDAs) or dietary reference intakes (DRIs).*

### 6. Health Considerations:
*Deficiencies in water-soluble vitamins can lead to a range of health problems, including beriberi (thiamine deficiency), pellagra (niacin deficiency), anemia (folate and B12 deficiency), and scurvy (vitamin C deficiency).*

### 7. Overconsumption:
*Water-soluble vitamins are generally considered safe, but excessive intake, especially through supplementation, can have adverse effects. Megadoses of certain B vitamins may lead to neurological symptoms.*

*In conclusion, water-soluble vitamins are vital for various bodily functions and need to be replenished regularly through a balanced diet. Including a variety of foods rich in these essential nutrients ensures that you receive the benefits of a healthy nervous system, immune function, energy metabolism, and overall well-being.*

# CHAPTER 8

## **Fat-Soluble Vitamins:** Essential Nutrients Stored in Fat

*Fat-soluble vitamins are a group of essential nutrients that are soluble in dietary fat and are stored in the body's fatty tissues. These vitamins include vitamin A, vitamin D, vitamin E, and vitamin K. Here's a comprehensive explanation of fat-soluble vitamins and their significance:*

### *1. Types of Fat-Soluble Vitamins:*

*Fat-soluble vitamins include:*

**Vitamin A: Exists in two main forms, retinol (found in animal sources) and provitamin A carotenoids (like beta-carotene, found in colorful fruits and vegetables).*

*Vitamin D: Comes in several forms, with vitamin D2 (ergocalciferol) from plant sources and vitamin D3 (cholecalciferol) primarily produced in the skin upon sun exposure.*

***Vitamin E: Refers to a group of compounds with antioxidant properties, including alpha-tocopherol.*

***Vitamin K: Exists in two forms, K1 (phylloquinone) and K2 (menaquinone), and is essential for blood clotting.*

## 2. Functions of Fat-Soluble Vitamins:

Fat-soluble vitamins serve various essential roles in the body:

**Vitamin A:** Essential for vision, immune function, and skin health.

**Vitamin D:** Critical for calcium absorption and bone health. It also plays a role in immune function.

**Vitamin E:** Acts as an antioxidant, protecting cells from oxidative damage.

**Vitamin K:** Essential for blood clotting and bone metabolism.

## 3. Solubility and Absorption:

Fat-soluble vitamins require the presence of dietary fat to be absorbed in the digestive system.

Unlike water-soluble vitamins, fat-soluble vitamins can be stored in the body's fatty tissues and liver. Excess amounts are not excreted as easily, and prolonged excessive intake can lead to toxicity.

## 4. Dietary Sources:

Fat-soluble vitamins are found in various foods, including:

**Vitamin A:** Sources include liver, dairy products, eggs, and orange and dark leafy green vegetables.

**Vitamin D:** Sunlight is a natural source, and dietary sources include fatty fish, fortified milk, and egg

**Vitamin E:** Found in nuts, seeds, vegetable oils, and some leafy greens.

**Vitamin K:** Abundant in leafy green vegetables, broccoli, and Brussels sprouts.

### 5. Recommended Intake:

Adequate intake of fat-soluble vitamins is specified in terms of recommended daily allowances (RDAs) or dietary reference intakes (DRIs), which vary based on age, gender, and specific health needs.

### 6. Health Considerations:

Deficiencies in fat-soluble vitamins can lead to various health issues, including night blindness (vitamin A deficiency), rickets (vitamin D deficiency), and clotting problems (vitamin K deficiency).
Overconsumption of fat-soluble vitamins can be harmful, particularly with vitamins A and D, as they can lead to toxicity and health problems.

### 7. Supplementation:

It's important to be cautious with fat-soluble vitamin supplements and take them only as recommended by a healthcare provider. Excessive intake from supplements can lead to toxicity.

In conclusion, **fat-soluble vitamins** are essential for numerous bodily functions and require dietary fat for absorption. A well-balanced diet that includes sources of these vitamins helps support healthy vision, bone health, immune function, and overall well-being while avoiding excessive intake to prevent potential toxicity.

# CHAPTER 9

## Minerals and Their Importance: Essential Nutrients for Health

Minerals are like the tiny superheroes of your body. They might not get as much attention as vitamins, but they play vital roles in keeping you healthy and functioning at your best. These essential minerals help with everything from building strong bones to keeping your heart beating regularly. Here's a look at some important minerals and what they do for you:

**Calcium:** Think of calcium as the building blocks for your bones and teeth. It's not just for kids; adults need it too to keep their bones strong. Calcium also helps with muscle function and blood clotting.

**Iron:** Iron is like a delivery person for oxygen. It helps carry oxygen to all the cells in your body. When you don't have enough iron, you can feel tired and weak.

**Sodium and Potassium:** These minerals are like the body's electricians. They help your nerves send signals and your muscles contract. They also keep the right balance of fluids in and around your cells.

**Magnesium:** Magnesium is involved in over 300 chemical reactions in your body. It's essential for muscle and nerve function, blood glucose control, and bone health.

**Phosphorus:** Phosphorus teams up with calcium to make your bones and teeth strong. It's also part of DNA and helps with energy metabolism.

**Zinc:** Zinc is like your body's repairman. It helps with wound healing, immune function, and making DNA.

**Copper:** Copper helps your body make collagen, a protein that's part of your skin, connective tissues, and blood vessels. It also acts as an antioxidant.

**Selenium:** Selenium works alongside other antioxidants to protect your cells from damage. It also plays a role in your thyroid function.

**Iodine:** Your thyroid gland needs iodine to make hormones that help regulate your metabolism and keep your body running smoothly.

**Fluoride:** Fluoride is a superhero for your teeth. It strengthens tooth enamel and helps protect them from cavities.

**Chromium:** Chromium is like a helper for insulin, the hormone that controls your blood sugar. It helps insulin do its job, which is essential for people with diabetes.

*These minerals are often found in the foods you eat, so a balanced diet is essential to make sure you get enough of them. When you get the right amount of these minerals, your body can work like a well-oiled machine, keeping you healthy and full of energy.*

# CHAPTER 10

## Digestive System Anatomy: How Your Body Processes Food

*The digestive system is like a complex network of tunnels, pipes, and factories that work together to process the food you eat. This system starts in your mouth and ends, well, at the other end. Let's take a journey through the anatomy of the digestive system:*

### 1. Mouth:
*It all begins here. Your teeth help break down food, and your tongue pushes it around.*
*Salivary glands produce saliva, which contains enzymes that start breaking down carbohydrates.*
*This is where you taste and chew your food, turning it into a mushy substance called bolus.*

### 2. Pharynx (Throat) and Esophagus:
*After you swallow, the bolus moves to your throat (pharynx) and then to the esophagus, a muscular tube.*
*The esophagus contracts to move the bolus downward, using a process called peristalsis.*

### 3. Stomach:

*The esophagus leads to the stomach, a J-shaped, muscular organ.*

*The stomach's strong acid and enzymes work to break down food further, creating a semi-liquid substance called chyme.*

### 4. Small Intestine:

*Chyme moves into the small intestine, a long, coiled tube.*

*The small intestine is where most of the absorption of nutrients happens. It has three parts: duodenum, jejunum, and ileum.*

*Tiny, finger-like structures called villi and microvilli inside the small intestine absorb nutrients and send them into your bloodstream.*

### 5. Liver:

*The liver, a large reddish-brown organ, sits on the right side of your abdomen.*

*It produces bile, which is essential for digesting fats. Bile is stored in the gallbladder.*

### 6. Gallbladder:

*The gallbladder is a small, greenish organ under the liver.*

*It stores bile and releases it into the small intestine when needed to help digest fats.*

### 7. Pancreas:

*The pancreas is a leaf-shaped gland located behind the stomach.*

*It releases digestive enzymes into the small intestine to further break down carbohydrates, proteins, and fats.*

### 8. Large Intestine (Colon):

*The leftover waste from the small intestine moves into the large intestine.*
*In the colon, water is absorbed from the waste, and it begins to solidify.*

### 9. Rectum and Anus:

*Finally, the now-formed waste is stored in the rectum until it's ready to leave your body.*
*When it's time to go, the anal sphincters open, and you have a bowel movement.*

### 10. Gut Microbiome:

*Throughout your digestive system, you have trillions of tiny microbes, known as the gut microbiome. These friendly bacteria help digest food, produce vitamins, and support your immune system.*

*The digestive system is an amazing and complex network of organs and tissues that work together to break down food, extract nutrients, and eliminate waste. Each part has a specific job, and if any part doesn't work properly, it can lead to digestive problems. So, taking care of your digestive system is crucial for overall health and well-being.*

# CHAPTER 11

## **Digestion and Absorption:** How Your Body Gets Nutrients from Food

*When you eat food, your body has to do some important work to turn that food into energy and building blocks for your body. This process is called digestion and absorption, and it's like a factory in your body that takes in raw materials (food) and turns them into useful products (nutrients).*

### *Step 1: The Mouth*

*It all starts in your mouth. When you take a bite of food, your teeth chew it up, and your saliva mixes with it. Saliva contains enzymes that begin breaking down carbohydrates in the food into smaller sugars. This is why your food starts to taste a bit sweet after you chew it for a while.*

### *Step 2: The Stomach*

*The food then travels to your stomach. Inside the stomach, there are strong acids and more enzymes. They work together to break down proteins into smaller pieces. Your stomach also mixes everything into a thick liquid called chyme. It's pretty acidic in there, which is why you don't feel so good if you have an empty stomach for too long.*

### Step 3: The Small Intestine

*Next stop, the small intestine. This is where most of the magic happens. The chyme from the stomach moves into the small intestine. Here, the pancreas and liver send in some special helpers. The pancreas releases enzymes that continue breaking down carbohydrates, proteins, and fats. The liver makes bile, which helps break down fats into tiny droplets. This makes it easier for enzymes to work on them.*

*As the nutrients get broken down, tiny finger-like structures called villi and microvilli in the lining of your small intestine absorb them. Think of these as little workers grabbing the small pieces of nutrients and sending them into your bloodstream, so they can be carried to the cells in your body.*

### Step 4: The Large Intestine

*After the small intestine, there's not much left for your body to use. So, the leftovers, like fiber and some water, move into your large intestine. The large intestine absorbs water and minerals, making sure you don't lose too much water when you go to the bathroom.*

### Step 5: Elimination

*Anything that your body can't use, like the parts of food that can't be digested, becomes waste. Your body sends this waste to your rectum and then out of your body through the anus. This is what we call a bowel movement or going to the bathroom.*

*So, in a nutshell, digestion and absorption are like a team effort involving your mouth, stomach, small intestine, and even your liver and pancreas. They work together to break down food and absorb the good stuff, which your body needs to stay healthy and full of energy.*

# CHAPTER 12

## Energy Balance and Metabolism: How Your Body Manages Energy

*Energy balance and metabolism are like the checks and balances of your body's energy needs. To stay healthy, your body needs the right amount of energy, which comes from the food you eat. Let's delve into the details of how your body manages energy:*

### 1. Energy Intake:
*It all starts with the food you eat. The energy in food is measured in calories. When you eat, you take in calories, which provide your body with energy.*
*Different foods have different calorie amounts. For example, fats have more calories per gram than carbohydrates or proteins.*

### 2. Digestion and Absorption:
*When you eat, your body digests the food, breaking it down into smaller molecules. Nutrients like carbohydrates, fats, and proteins are absorbed into your bloodstream from the digestive system.*

### 3. Metabolism:

Your body's metabolism is like a set of chemical reactions that happen inside your cells. These reactions are responsible for turning the nutrients from food into energy.

Metabolism includes two main processes:

**Catabolism:** This process breaks down larger molecules into smaller ones, releasing energy. For example, breaking down glucose for energy.

**Anabolism:** This process builds larger molecules from smaller ones, consuming energy. For example, using energy to create new proteins.

### 4. Energy Expenditure:

Your body spends energy on various activities and functions:

**Basal Metabolic Rate (BMR):** This is the energy your body needs to perform basic functions like breathing, maintaining body temperature, and repairing cells. BMR makes up a significant part of your daily energy expenditure.

**Physical Activity:** Any movement, from walking to exercising, burns calories. The more active you are, the more energy you use.

**Thermic Effect of Food (TEF):** Digesting, absorbing, and storing the nutrients from food also requires energy.

**Non-Exercise Activity Thermogenesis (NEAT):** Everyday activities like fidgeting, standing, and even talking consume energy.

**Adaptive Thermogenesis:** In some situations, your body may increase energy expenditure, like when you're exposed to cold temperatures.

### 5. Energy Balance:

Maintaining a healthy weight and energy balance is about matching energy intake (calories from food) with energy expenditure (calories burned through metabolism and activities).

Three scenarios can occur:

**Positive Energy Balance:** When you consume more calories than you burn, you gain weight.

**Negative Energy Balance:** When you burn more calories than you consume, you lose weight.

**Maintenance Energy Balance:** When calorie intake equals caloric expenditure, your weight remains stable.

### 6. Hormones and Regulation:

Hormones like insulin, glucagon, and leptin play a role in regulating energy balance and metabolism.

For example, insulin helps control blood sugar levels and store excess energy as fat, while leptin signals your brain to control appetite.

### 7. Factors Influencing Energy Balance:

Factors like genetics, age, gender, and muscle mass can affect your BMR.

Psychological factors, such as stress and emotional eating, can influence food intake.

### 8. Health Implications:

Maintaining a healthy energy balance is crucial for overall health. Positive energy balance can lead to

*weight gain and obesity, while negative energy balance can result in weight loss.*
*Proper energy balance is essential for maintaining a healthy weight and preventing various chronic diseases.*

*Understanding energy balance and metabolism is key to making informed choices about your diet, exercise, and overall health. It's a delicate equilibrium that your body strives to maintain to keep you feeling your best.*

# CHAPTER 13

## Body Mass Index (BMI): A Simple Measure of Health

*BMI is a straightforward tool that helps you understand whether your weight is in a healthy range for your height. It's a helpful way to gauge your overall health, but remember, it's just one part of the bigger picture.*

### 1. Calculation:
*BMI is calculated by dividing your weight in kilograms by your height in meters squared. The formula looks like this: BMI = weight (kg) / (height (m))^2. Or, if you use pounds and inches: BMI = (weight (lb) / (height (in)^2)) x 703.*

### 2. BMI Categories:
*Based on your BMI score, you fall into one of several categories:*
*Underweight: BMI less than 18.5*
*Normal weight: BMI between 18.5 and 24.9*
*Overweight: BMI between 25 and 29.9*
*Obesity:*
*Class I: BMI between 30 and 34.9*
*Class II: BMI between 35 and 39.9*

*Class III (Severe Obesity): BMI 40 or higher*

### 3. What BMI Tells You:

BMI provides a general idea of your body's weight relative to your height. It's often used to identify potential health risks associated with being underweight, overweight, or obese.

A **"normal"** BMI suggests you're at a healthy weight for your height. However, it doesn't consider factors like muscle mass, bone density, and where your body stores fat.

### 4. Limitations:

BMI is a useful tool, but it has limitations. It doesn't account for variations in muscle mass, body composition, or other factors like age and sex.

Athletes or people with high muscle mass may have a high BMI, even if they're not overweight.

### 5. Health Implications:

High BMI values are associated with a higher risk of health issues such as heart disease, diabetes, and certain cancers.

Low BMI can indicate malnutrition or other health problems.

### 6. Considerations:

It's essential to remember that BMI is just one part of assessing your health. Other factors like waist circumference, body composition, and lifestyle habits are crucial in determining overall well-being.

*Always consult a healthcare professional for a comprehensive health assessment.*

### 7. Using BMI Wisely:

*Don't focus on BMI alone. It's a starting point, not the final word on your health.*

*If your BMI suggests you're underweight, overweight, or obese, consult with a healthcare provider to evaluate your overall health and discuss strategies for improvement.*

*In summary, BMI is a simple tool that gives you a quick estimate of your body's weight status. It's useful for identifying potential health risks associated with weight, but it's just one piece of the puzzle. To understand your overall health, consider other factors and consult a healthcare professional for personalized guidance.*

# CHAPTER 14

## **Understanding Calories:** What You Need to Know About Energy

*Calories are the units of energy your body uses to function. Whether you're running a marathon or simply breathing, your body requires energy, measured in calories, to perform these activities. Here's a detailed explanation of calories and how they affect your daily life:*

### *1. What Are Calories?*

*A calorie is a unit of measurement for energy. Specifically, it's the amount of heat required to raise the temperature of one gram of water by one degree Celsius. In the context of food and nutrition, we use kilocalories, often referred to as "calories."*

### *2. Energy Intake:*

*When you eat, you're taking in calories from the food and beverages you consume. The number of calories you ingest provides your body with the energy it needs to carry out daily functions and activities.*

### *3. Energy Expenditure:*

*Your body burns calories through various processes, including:*

**Basal Metabolic Rate (BMR):** *The energy your body needs at rest to maintain basic functions like breathing and cell repair.*

**Physical Activity:** *The calories burned during exercise, work, and daily activities.*

**Thermic Effect of Food (TEF):** *The energy required to digest, absorb, and metabolize the nutrients in the food you eat.*

**Non-Exercise Activity Thermogenesis (NEAT):** *The calories expended during non-exercise activities like fidgeting or standing.*

### *4. Energy Balance:*

*Achieving a balance between the calories you consume and the calories you burn is crucial for maintaining your weight.*

*If you consume more calories than your body needs, you'll gain weight.*

*If you consume fewer calories than your body needs, you'll lose weight.*

*If your calorie intake matches your energy expenditure, your weight remains stable.*

### *5. Daily Caloric Needs:*

*Your daily calorie needs are influenced by factors like age, gender, weight, activity level, and metabolic rate.*

*To estimate your daily calorie needs, you can use tools like the Harris-Benedict Equation or consult with a healthcare professional.*

### 6. Macronutrients and Calories:

*Different macronutrients provide different amounts of calories per gram:*

**Carbohydrates**: *Provide about 4 calories per gram.*
**Proteins:** *Also provide about 4 calories per gram.*
**Fats:** *Provide around 9 calories per gram.*
**Alcohol:** *Provides about 7 calories per gram.*

### 7. Caloric Content of Food:

*The nutritional labels on food packages display the calorie content per serving, helping you make informed dietary choices.*

### 8. Caloric Surplus and Deficit:

*A caloric surplus occurs when you consume more calories than you burn. It leads to weight gain.*

*A caloric deficit happens when you burn more calories than you consume. It results in weight loss.*

### 9. Health Implications:

*The quality of calories you consume is as important as the quantity. A diet rich in nutrient-dense foods is essential for overall health.*

### 10. Balancing Calories:

*Striking the right balance between calorie intake and expenditure is key to achieving and maintaining a healthy weight.*

It's important to focus on a well-rounded diet, physical activity, and a sustainable approach to managing calories for long-term health.

Understanding calories is essential for making informed dietary and lifestyle choices. By finding the right balance, you can fuel your body effectively, maintain a healthy weight, and support your overall well-being.

# CHAPTER 15

## Nutritional Needs at Different Life Stages: Tailoring Your Diet for Health

*Nutritional needs change throughout life. It's like having a customized meal plan for each stage. Here's an overview of how nutritional requirements evolve from infancy to old age:*

### 1. Infancy (0-2 years):
**Breast Milk or Formula:** *Babies rely on breast milk or infant formula for optimal nutrition. Breast milk offers essential nutrients and antibodies for a strong start.*
**Introduction of Solid Foods:** *Around 6 months, infants begin eating solid foods, starting with pureed fruits and vegetables and gradually incorporating other foods.*
**Nutrient Focus:** *Infants need nutrients like iron, calcium, and healthy fats to support rapid growth and brain development.*

### 2. Childhood (3-12 years):
**Balanced Diet:** *As kids grow, they need a balanced diet rich in fruits, vegetables, whole grains, lean proteins, and dairy for bone health.*

**Adequate Calcium:** *Calcium is crucial for building strong bones. Milk, yogurt, and fortified foods are excellent sources.*

**Limit Added Sugars:** *Limiting added sugars is essential to prevent childhood obesity and dental issues.*

### 3. Adolescence (13-18 years):

**Nutrient-Dense Foods:** *Teens need nutrient-dense foods to fuel growth spurts and meet increased energy demands.*

**Iron and Calcium:** *Adolescents, especially girls, need extra iron for growth and development. Calcium intake is vital for bone health.*

**Hydration:** *Staying well-hydrated is crucial, especially for active teens.*

### 4. Young Adulthood (19-30 years):

**Balanced Diet:** *Young adults should maintain a balanced diet with an emphasis on whole, unprocessed foods.*

**Folate and Iron:** *For women of childbearing age, folate is crucial for preventing birth defects. Iron is still essential.*

**Healthy Fats:** *Incorporate healthy fats like those from avocados, nuts, and fatty fish.*

### 5. Middle Adulthood (31-50 years):

**Lean Proteins:** *Lean proteins support muscle maintenance and bone health.*

**Fiber:** *Adequate fiber intake aids digestion and may reduce the risk of chronic diseases.*

*Folate and Calcium:* Continue to focus on these nutrients, especially for women.

### 6. Late Adulthood (51+ years):
*Calcium and Vitamin D:* Bone health becomes a priority, so calcium and vitamin D are essential.
*B Vitamins:* B vitamins, including B12, become more important as absorption may decrease with age.
*Protein:* Maintaining muscle mass and strength becomes crucial.

### 7. Pregnancy and Lactation:
*Folate:* Folate helps prevent birth defects, so it's essential during pregnancy.
*Iron:* Iron supports increased blood volume and fetal growth.
*Calcium and Vitamin D:* These nutrients are vital for both the mother's and baby's bone health.
*Hydration:* Staying well-hydrated is essential for pregnant and lactating women.

### 8. Older Adults (65+ years):
*Protein:*Maintaining muscle mass and strength is vital.
*B Vitamins:* Adequate B12 intake is crucial for seniors.
*Fiber and Hydration:* Fiber aids digestion, and staying well-hydrated helps manage dehydration risks.

### 9. Special Diets:
People with specific dietary requirements, like vegetarians or those with food allergies, should adapt their diets to meet nutritional needs.

*Nutritional needs vary by age and life stage. Meeting these changing requirements with a balanced diet helps support growth, health, and well-being throughout life. Consulting a healthcare provider or registered dietitian can offer personalized guidance for specific life stages or dietary concerns.*

# CHAPTER 16

## Nutrition for Children: Building Healthy Habits for Life

*Children's nutrition is essential for their growth, development, and overall well-being. Proper nutrition sets the stage for a healthy life. Here's a comprehensive explanation of nutrition for children:*

### 1. Balanced Diet:

*Children need a balanced diet that includes a variety of foods from different food groups:*

**Fruits and Vegetables:** *These provide vitamins, minerals, and fiber. Encourage colorful options.*

*****Whole Grains:** *Whole grains offer essential carbohydrates and fiber. Choose whole wheat bread, brown rice, and whole-grain pasta.*

**Proteins:** *Protein sources include lean meats, poultry, fish, beans, lentils, nuts, and seeds.*

**Dairy:** *Offer dairy products like milk, yogurt, and cheese for calcium and vitamin D.*

### 2. Portion Control:

*Appropriate portion sizes are crucial. Children's portion sizes should be smaller than those for adults but adjusted for their age and activity level.*

### 3. Snacking:

Snacks can be part of a healthy diet if they consist of nutritious options like fruit, yogurt, or whole-grain crackers. Limit sugary snacks and beverages.

### 4. Hydration:

Encourage water as the primary beverage. Limit sugary drinks, such as soda and fruit juices.

For active children, especially in hot Weather, sports drinks can help replenish electrolytes lost through sweating.

### 5. Meal Timing:

Regular meals and snacks help maintain energy levels and prevent overeating. Children often need small, frequent meals.

### 6. Micronutrients:

Children require essential vitamins and minerals, such as vitamin D for bone health, iron for growth, and calcium for strong bones.

A balanced diet usually provides these nutrients, but pediatrician-recommended supplements may be necessary in some cases.

### 7. Dietary Restrictions:

Be mindful of any dietary restrictions due to allergies or cultural preferences. Ensure your child gets the nutrients they need through alternative food sources.

### 8. Encouraging Healthy Eating Habits:

Model healthy eating behaviors as children learn by example.
Involve children in meal planning and preparation to make them more interested in their food.

### 9. Growth and Development:

Nutrient requirements vary as children grow. Be aware of growth spurts and adjust portion sizes and food choices accordingly.

### 10. Special Diets:

Children with specific dietary requirements, like vegetarians or those with food allergies, need carefully planned diets to meet their nutritional needs.

### 11. Limit Sugars and Processed Foods:

Excess sugar intake can lead to weight gain and dental problems. Minimize the consumption of sugary snacks and processed foods.

### 12. Monitor Screen Time:

Excessive screen time may lead to poor eating habits. Limit screen time and encourage physical activity.

### 13. Food Safety:

Ensure food safety to prevent foodborne illnesses. Teach children the importance of washing hands before meals.

### 14. Consult a Pediatrician:

*Regular check-ups with a pediatrician can help track growth and nutritional needs. Discuss any concerns about your child's diet or growth.*

**15. Be Patient:**
*Children may be picky eaters. It may take multiple exposures to new foods before they develop a taste for them.*

*Nutrition is a fundamental part of childhood health and development. By providing a balanced and nutritious diet, encouraging healthy eating habits, and seeking professional guidance when needed, you can set your child on a path to a lifetime of good health.*

# CHAPTER 17

## Nutrition for Adolescents: Fueling Growth and Health

*Adolescence is a critical stage of life when growth and development are at their peak. Proper nutrition during this period is essential for physical, cognitive, and emotional well-being. Here's a comprehensive explanation of nutrition for adolescents:*

### 1. Balanced Diet:

*Adolescents need a balanced diet rich in essential nutrients. Their nutritional needs include:*

***Proteins:*** *Important for growth and muscle development. Sources include lean meats, poultry, fish, beans, and nuts.*

***Calcium:*** *Crucial for bone health. Dairy products, fortified foods, and leafy greens are good sources.*

***Iron:*** *Required for the expansion of blood volume and muscle development. Include red meat, beans, and fortified cereals.*

***Folate:*** *Essential for cell division and growth. Found in green leafy vegetables and fortified grains.*

***Whole Grains:*** *Provide complex carbohydrates and fiber for energy and digestion.*

**Fruits and Vegetables:** *Rich in vitamins, minerals, and antioxidants. Encourage a variety of colorful options.*

**Dairy or Dairy Alternatives:** *Offer calcium and vitamin D for bone health.*

### 2. Protein Needs:

*Adolescents have increased protein needs due to growth. Encourage the inclusion of lean protein sources in meals and snacks.*

### 3. Hydration:

*Adequate water intake is vital, especially for active adolescents. Encourage water as the primary beverage and limit sugary drinks.*

### 4. Snacking:

*Healthy snacks can be part of an adolescent's diet. Opt for nutrient-dense options like fruit, yogurt, or nuts.*

### 5. Balanced Meals:

*Regular, balanced meals help maintain energy levels and provide necessary nutrients.*

### 6. Special Diets:

*Adolescents with dietary restrictions, such as vegetarians or those with food allergies, require well-planned diets to meet their nutritional needs.*

### 7. Growth and Development:

*Adolescents experience rapid growth and development. Ensure they have enough calories to support this growth while maintaining a healthy weight.*

### 8. Limit Sugars and Processed Foods:
*Reduce the consumption of sugary snacks and processed foods to prevent weight gain and promote overall health.*

### 9. Physical Active
*Encourage regular physical activity to support growth, strengthen muscles and bones, and maintain a healthy weight.*

### 10. Body Image and Self-Esteem:
*Adolescence is a time when body image and self-esteem become significant. Promote a healthy body image and emphasize the importance of self-acceptance and self-worth.*

### 11. Monitor Screen Time:
*Excessive screen time can lead to sedentary behavior and unhealthy eating habits. Set limits on screen time and encourage outdoor activities.*

### 12. Be Patient:
*Adolescents may experiment with food and eating habits. Be patient and provide guidance on making healthy choices.*

### 13. Consult a Healthcare Provider:

*Regular check-ups with a healthcare provider can help monitor growth, nutritional needs, and overall health. Discuss any concerns about dietary habits, growth, or development.*

## 14. Nutritional Education:
*Provide adolescents with the knowledge and skills to make informed food choices and develop a healthy relationship with food.*

## 15. Mental Health:
*Promote mental well-being and address any mental health concerns that may impact eating habits and overall health.*

*Adolescence is a crucial time for establishing lifelong eating habits and maintaining physical and emotional health. By offering a balanced diet, fostering a positive body image, encouraging physical activity, and addressing any specific dietary needs, you can help adolescents navigate this period with confidence and good health.*

# CHAPTER 18

## Nutrition for Adults: Nourishing Your Health and Well-Being

*Nutrition remains a fundamental pillar of health throughout adulthood. As we age, our nutritional needs change, and making informed choices is crucial for maintaining well-being. Here's a comprehensive explanation of nutrition for adults:*

### 1. Balanced Diet:

*A balanced diet is the foundation of good nutrition. Adults should aim to include a variety of foods from different food groups, including:*

**Fruits and Vegetables:** *Rich in vitamins, minerals, and fiber.*

**Whole Grains:** *Provide complex carbohydrates and fiber for sustained energy and digestive health.*

**Proteins:** *Essential for muscle maintenance and overall health. Sources include lean meats, poultry, fish, beans, and nuts.*

**Dairy or Dairy Alternatives:** *Offer calcium for bone health.*

 **Healthy Fats:**** *Include sources of healthy fats like avocados, nuts, and fatty fish.*

## 2. Portion Control:
*Be mindful of portion sizes to manage calorie intake and maintain a healthy weight.*

## 3. Hydration:
*Staying well-hydrated is crucial for overall health. Water is the best choice, but herbal teas and unsweetened beverages are also suitable.*

## 4. Snacking:
*Healthy snacks can be part of a balanced diet. Opt for nutrient-dense options like fruit, yogurt, or raw vegetables.*

## 5. Fiber Intake:
*Adequate fiber intake supports digestive health and may reduce the risk of chronic diseases.*

## 6. Limit Sugars and Processed Foods:
*Minimize the consumption of sugary snacks and processed foods, as they can contribute to weight gain and health issues.*

## 7. Nutrient-Dense Choices:
*Focus on nutrient-dense foods that offer a high level of nutrients relative to their calorie content.*

## 8. Dietary Restrictions:

Adults with specific dietary requirements, such as vegetarians or those with food allergies, should adapt their diets to meet their nutritional needs.

### 9. Special Diets:
Special diets may be necessary for medical conditions or specific health goals, such as heart-healthy or diabetes-friendly diets.

### 10. Portion Control:
Monitoring portion sizes helps maintain a healthy weight and prevent overeating.

### 11. Balanced Meals:
Consistent, balanced meals ensure the intake of essential nutrients and maintain energy levels.

### 12. Limit Alcohol:
If you consume alcohol, do so in moderation. Excessive alcohol consumption can lead to various health issues.

### 13. Physical Activity:
Regular physical activity supports muscle and bone health, weight management, and overall well-being.

### 14. Screen Time:
Limit screen time and prioritize face-to-face social interactions to promote mental well-being and reduce sedentary behavior.

### 15. Mental Health:

Mental health plays a crucial role in overall well-being. Manage stress and seek help for any mental health concerns.

### 16. Regular Health Check-Ups:
Regular check-ups with a healthcare provider are important for monitoring overall health, addressing specific dietary needs, and discussing any concerns.

### 17. Nutritional Education:
Stay informed about the latest nutrition research and guidelines to make informed food choices.

### 18. Hydration:
Water is essential for bodily functions. Ensure proper hydration throughout the day.

### 19. Balance and Moderation:
Finding balance in your diet and exercising moderation is key to maintaining a healthy relationship with food.

### 20. Meal Preparation:
Preparing meals at home allows you to control ingredients and make healthier choices.

Nutrition remains a cornerstone of health and well-being throughout adulthood. By making informed dietary choices, staying physically active, and addressing specific nutritional needs, adults can maintain good health and enjoy a high quality of life.

# CHAPTER 19

## Nutrition for Seniors: Nourishing Health and Well-Being in the Golden Years

*As we age, our nutritional needs change, and paying attention to dietary choices becomes even more important for maintaining health and well-being. Here's a comprehensive explanation of nutrition for seniors:*

### 1. Balanced Diet:
*A balanced diet is essential, but specific nutritional needs may vary. Seniors should focus on a variety of foods from different groups, including:*
**Fruits and Vegetables:** *These provide essential vitamins, minerals, and fiber.*
**Whole Grains:** *For complex carbohydrates and fiber to support digestion.*
**Proteins:** *Crucial for muscle maintenance and overall health. Sources include lean meats, poultry, fish, beans, and nuts.*
**Dairy or Dairy Alternatives:** *Offer calcium for bone health.*
**Healthy Fats:** *Include sources of healthy fats like avocados, nuts, and fatty fish.*

### 2. Portion Control:

Seniors may require fewer calories, so portion control helps prevent overeating and weight gain.

### 3. Hydration:
Proper hydration is crucial for seniors. Encourage adequate water intake to prevent dehydration.

### 4. Fiber Intake:
Adequate fiber supports digestive health and may reduce the risk of chronic diseases.

### 5. Nutrient-Dense Choices:
Focus on nutrient-dense foods that provide a high level of nutrients relative to their calorie content.

### 6. Limit Sugars and Processed Foods:
Minimize the consumption of sugary snacks and processed foods, as they can contribute to health issues.

### 7. Dietary Restrictions:
Seniors with specific dietary needs, such as vegetarians or those with food allergies, should adapt their diets accordingly.

### 8. Special Diets:
Special diets may be necessary for medical conditions, such as heart-healthy or diabetes-friendly diets.

### 9. Balanced Meals:

*Consistent, balanced meals ensure the intake of essential nutrients and maintain energy levels.*

### 10. Vitamin and Mineral Supplementation:
*Some seniors may require supplements for specific nutrients like vitamin B12, vitamin D, or calcium. Consult a healthcare provider for guidance.*

### 11. Alcohol and Medication Interactions:
*Be aware of potential interactions between alcohol and medications. Consult a healthcare provider if you have concerns.*

### 12. Physical Activity:
*Regular physical activity helps maintain muscle and bone health, manage weight, and promote overall well-being.*

### 13. Screen Time:
*Limit screen time and engage in social activities to maintain mental and emotional health.*

### 14. Mental Health:
*Prioritize mental health by managing stress and seeking help for any mental health concerns.*

### 15. Regular Health Check-Ups:
*Regular check-ups with a healthcare provider are essential for monitoring overall health, addressing specific dietary needs, and discussing any concerns.*

### *16. Hydration:*

*Seniors may have a reduced sensation of thirst, so it's crucial to stay well-hydrated.*

### 17. Balance and Stability:

*Include exercises that enhance balance and stability to reduce the risk of falls and injuries.*

### 18. Oral Health:

*Maintain good oral hygiene and dental health. Chewing difficulties can affect food choices.*

### *19. Social Engagement:*

*Staying socially active can improve mental and emotional well-being.*

### *20. Independence and Autonomy:*

*Encourage seniors to maintain autonomy and independence in food choices, when possible, to ensure a sense of control.*

*Nutrition plays a pivotal role in senior health and well-being. By staying informed about dietary choices, engaging in physical and social activities, addressing specific nutritional needs, and seeking regular healthcare check-ups, seniors can enjoy a high quality of life in their golden years.*

# CHAPTER 20

## Nutritional Needs During Pregnancy: Nourishing for Two

*Pregnancy is a unique and transformative period in a woman's life. Proper nutrition during pregnancy is crucial for the health and development of both the mother and the baby. Here's a comprehensive explanation of the nutritional needs during pregnancy:*

### 1. Balanced Diet:

*A balanced diet is the foundation of a healthy pregnancy. It should include a variety of foods from different food groups, such as:*

***Fruits and Vegetables:*** *Rich in vitamins, minerals, and fiber. A variety of colorful options is encouraged.*

***Whole Grains:*** *Provide complex carbohydrates and fiber for energy and digestion.*

***Proteins:*** *Essential for fetal growth and overall health. Include lean meats, poultry, fish, beans, and nuts.*

***Dairy or Dairy Alternatives:*** *Offer calcium for the baby's bone development.*

**Healthy Fats:** *Include sources of healthy fats like avocados, nuts, and fatty fish.*

## 2. Increased Calories:
*During pregnancy, extra calories are needed to support the growing baby. The recommended calorie increase varies, but typically, an additional 300-500 calories per day are suggested.*

## 3. Protein Needs:
*Protein is essential for the baby's growth and should be included in every meal.*

## 4. Folate and Iron:
*Folate is essential for preventing neural tube defects. Iron is necessary to support the increased blood volume.*
*Prenatal supplements often contain these nutrients, but they should be obtained through food as well.*

## 5. Hydration:
*Staying well-hydrated is vital during pregnancy. Water is the best choice, but herbal teas and unsweetened beverages are also suitable.*

## 6. Nutrient-Dense Choices:
*Opt for nutrient-dense foods that offer high nutritional value for the calories consumed.*

## 7. Limit Sugars and Processed Foods:

*Minimize the consumption of sugary snacks and processed foods, as they can contribute to weight gain and health issues.*

### 8. Fiber Intake:
*Adequate fiber intake supports digestion and may help with common pregnancy discomforts like constipation.*

### 9. Special Dietary Considerations:
*Women with specific dietary restrictions, such as vegetarians or those with food allergies, should adapt their diets to meet their nutritional needs.*

### 10. Meal Timing:
*Regular meals and snacks help maintain energy levels and provide essential nutrients.*

### 11. Vitamin and Mineral Supplementation:
*Prenatal vitamins are often recommended to ensure that mothers meet their nutritional needs. Consult with a healthcare provider for guidance on which supplements are appropriate.*

### 12. Limit Caffeine and Alcohol:
*Limit caffeine and avoid alcohol during pregnancy, as both can have adverse effects on the baby.*

### 13. Consult a Healthcare Provider:
*Regular prenatal check-ups are essential for monitoring the baby's development and addressing specific dietary needs.*

### 14. Morning Sickness:

If morning sickness is a concern, seek guidance from a healthcare provider on managing symptoms and maintaining proper nutrition.

### 15. Food Safety:

Be vigilant about food safety to prevent foodborne illnesses, which can be more dangerous during pregnancy.

### 16. Mental Health:

Pregnancy can be a time of emotional ups and downs. Pay attention to mental health and seek support when needed.

### 17. Balanced Weight Gain:

Achieving a balanced weight gain is important. Consult with a healthcare provider for personalized guidance.

Nutrition during pregnancy is a pivotal factor in the health and well-being of both the mother and the baby. By following a balanced diet, staying hydrated, taking supplements as needed, and seeking regular prenatal care, expectant mothers can provide the best possible start for their child's life.

# CHAPTER 21

## Nutritional Needs During Lactation: Nourishing for Two

*Lactation is a critical period when a mother's body provides all the nutrients her baby needs through breast milk. Proper nutrition during this time is essential for the health and development of the baby. Here's a comprehensive explanation of the nutritional needs during lactation:*

### 1. Balanced Diet:

*A balanced diet is crucial for lactating mothers. It should include a variety of foods from different food groups, such as:*

**Fruits and Vegetables:** *Rich in vitamins, minerals, and fiber. A variety of colorful options is encouraged.*

**Whole Grains:** *Provide complex carbohydrates and fiber for energy and digestion.*

**Proteins:** *Essential for milk production and overall health. Include lean meats, poultry, fish, beans, and nuts.*

**Dairy or Dairy Alternatives:** *Offer calcium for both the baby and the mother's bone health.*

**Healthy Fats:** *Include sources of healthy fats like avocados, nuts, and fatty fish.*

### 2. Increased Calories:

Lactating mothers require additional calories to support milk production. The exact calorie increase varies, but it's typically recommended to add around 500 calories per day.

### 3. Protein Needs:

Adequate protein intake is necessary for milk production and overall health.

### 4. Hydration:

Staying well-hydrated is vital during lactation. Proper hydration supports milk production and helps prevent dehydration.

### 5. Nutrient-Dense Choices:

Opt for nutrient-dense foods to ensure that both the mother and baby receive the essential nutrients they need.

### 6. Limit Sugars and Processed Foods:

Minimize the consumption of sugary snacks and processed foods, as they can contribute to weight gain and health issues.

### 7. Fiber Intake:

Adequate fiber intake supports digestion and may help with postpartum recovery.

### 8. Vitamin and Mineral Supplementation:

Prenatal vitamins are often recommended for lactating mothers to ensure that they meet their nutritional needs. Consult with a healthcare provider for guidance on supplements.

### 9. Caffeine and Alcohol:

Limit caffeine intake and avoid alcohol during lactation, as both substances can have effects on the baby.

### 10. Consult a Healthcare Provider:

Regular check-ups with a healthcare provider are essential to monitor the baby's development and the mother's health.

### 11. Food Safety:

Be vigilant about food safety to prevent foodborne illnesses, which can affect both the mother and the baby.

### 12. Mental Health:

Lactation can be a time of emotional ups and downs. Pay attention to mental health and seek support when needed.

### 13. Listen to Your Body:

Lactating mothers should pay attention to their bodies and hunger cues. Eating when hungry and resting when needed are essential for milk production and self-care.

*Lactation is a vital time for a mother to provide the best possible start for her baby's life. By following a balanced diet, staying hydrated, taking supplements as recommended, and seeking regular postpartum care, nursing mothers can support their baby's growth and development while maintaining their own health and well-being.*

# CHAPTER 22

## Macronutrient Ratios in Diets: Finding the Right Balance:

*Macronutrients are the primary components of the human diet, and the ratio in which we consume them plays a significant role in our overall health and well-being. Here's an explanation of macronutrients and the importance of finding the right balance in your diet:*

### 1. Carbohydrates:

*   **Role:*  Carbohydrates are the body's primary source of energy. They provide fuel for physical and mental activities.*
*   **Recommended Ratio:*  Around 45-65% of total daily calories should come from carbohydrates.*
*   **Sources:*  Whole grains, fruits, vegetables, legumes, and starchy foods.*

### 2. Proteins:

*   **Role:* Proteins are essential for growth, tissue repair, and the production of enzymes and hormones.*
*   **Recommended Ratio:* Approximately 10-35% of daily calories should come from protein.*
*   **Sources:*  Lean meats, poultry, fish, beans, lentils, dairy, and plant-based protein sources.*

### 3. Fats:

**Role:** Fats provide long-lasting energy, support cell growth, and aid in the absorption of fat-soluble vitamins.

**Recommended Ratio:** About 20-35% of daily calories should come from fats.

**Sources:** Healthy fats from avocados, nuts, seeds, olive oil, and fatty fish. Limit saturated and trans fats.

### 4. Finding the Right Balance:

The ideal macronutrient ratio depends on individual factors such as age, activity level, and health goals.

A balanced diet typically includes a higher percentage of carbohydrates for energy, moderate protein for muscle maintenance, and healthy fats for overall well-being.

### 5. Dietary Goals:

Tailor your macronutrient ratios to specific dietary goals:

**Weight Loss:** Reducing carbohydrate intake and increasing protein and fiber can aid in weight management.

**Muscle Building:** A higher protein intake is essential for those focused on muscle development.

**Heart Health:** Reducing saturated and trans fats while increasing healthy fats can improve cardiovascular health.

**Steady Energy:** Consuming complex carbohydrates provides steady, sustained energy throughout the day.

### 6. Individualized Needs:

Everyone's dietary requirements are unique. Consider your age, gender, activity level, and health conditions when determining your macronutrient ratios.

### 7. Balanced Diet:

A balanced diet typically consists of a variety of foods from all food groups, ensuring an adequate intake of macronutrients and micronutrients.

### 8. Dietary Trends:

Various dietary trends, like low-carb or high-protein diets, focus on specific macronutrient ratios. Choose a plan that aligns with your goals and consult a healthcare provider if you have concerns.

### 9. Moderation:

Avoid extremes. Extreme diets that restrict or overemphasize certain macronutrients may lead to imbalances and nutritional deficiencies.

### 10. Monitoring and Adaptation:

Pay attention to how your body responds to your diet. Regular monitoring and adjustments are key to finding the right macronutrient balance for you.

Balancing macronutrients in your diet is a dynamic process that should align with your health goals and lifestyle. It's essential to find a ratio that supports your individual needs, provides the necessary nutrients for overall health, and helps you achieve your dietary and *fitness objectives. Consulting a registered dietitian or healthcare provider can offer personalized guidance.*

# CHAPTER 23

## The Mediterranean Diet: A Healthy and Flavorful Lifestyle

*The Mediterranean diet is a well-known and widely acclaimed eating pattern that originated in the Mediterranean region. It's renowned for its numerous health benefits, delectable flavors, and overall focus on well-being. Here's a comprehensive explanation of the Mediterranean diet:*

### 1. Key Principles:
**The Mediterranean diet emphasizes several key principles:**

*Abundant consumption of fruits and vegetables.*
*Whole grains as the primary source of carbohydrates.*
*Healthy fats, especially olive oil.*
*Moderate consumption of fish and poultry.*
*Limited red meat intake.*
*Incorporation of legumes, nuts, and seeds.*
*Use of herbs and spices for flavor instead of salt.*
*Moderate wine consumption, usually during meals.*
*Social and physical activity as essential components of a healthy lifestyle.*

### 2. Nutritional Components:
*The Mediterranean diet is rich in several important nutrients:*

**Healthy Fats:** *Olive oil is a staple, providing monounsaturated fats that support heart health.*

**Fruits and Vegetables:** *Abundant sources of vitamins, minerals, fiber, and antioxidants.*

**Whole Grains:** *Whole wheat, barley, and bulgur are common sources of complex carbohydrates and fiber.*

**Proteins:** *Fish, particularly fatty fish like salmon and mackerel, provide omega-3 fatty acids. Legumes, nuts, and seeds are sources of plant-based protein.*

**Moderate Wine Consumption:** *Red wine, when consumed in moderation, may offer cardiovascular benefits due to its polyphenol content.*

### 3. Health Benefits:

*The Mediterranean diet is associated with numerous health advantages, including:*

*Reduced risk of heart disease and stroke.*

*Improved weight management and reduced risk of obesity.*

*Lower risk of type 2 diabetes.*

*Enhanced cognitive function and reduced risk of Alzheimer's disease.*

*Lower rates of certain cancers.*

*Better management of chronic conditions like hypertension and high cholesterol.*

*Improved longevity and overall well-being.*

### 4. Lifestyle Factors:

*The Mediterranean diet is not just about food. It also promotes a holistic approach to well-being:*

**Social Connections:** *The Mediterranean lifestyle often involves communal meals, promoting social connections and emotional well-being.*

**Physical Activity:** *Regular physical activity, often integrated into daily life, is a core part of the Mediterranean lifestyle.*

**Mindfulness:** *Savoring meals and appreciating the flavors and company is central to this diet.*

**Relaxation:** *Reducing stress and taking time to relax are significant aspects of the Mediterranean way of life.*

## 5. Sustainability:

*The Mediterranean diet is often considered an environmentally friendly choice due to its reliance on seasonal, locally sourced ingredients.*

## 6. Practical Tips:

*To follow the Mediterranean diet, consider these practical tips:*

*Use olive oil as your primary source of fat.*

*Increase your intake of fruits, vegetables, and whole grains.*

*Opt for fish and poultry over red meat.*

*include legumes, nuts, and seeds in your meals.*

*Use herbs and spices for flavor.*

*Enjoy a glass of red wine in moderation if you choose to drink alcohol.*

*Engage in physical activity and make time for relaxation and social connections.*

The Mediterranean diet is a delicious and sustainable way of eating that promotes numerous health benefits. By embracing its principles, you can enjoy flavorful, wholesome meals while supporting your overall well-being. It's a lifestyle that embodies the joy of eating, social connection, and a profound appreciation for life.

# CHAPTER 24

## The Keto Diet: Understanding Ketosis and Low-Carb Living.

*The ketogenic diet, often referred to as the **"keto"** diet, is a low-carbohydrate, high-fat eating plan designed to induce a state of ketosis in the body. Ketosis is a metabolic state where the body primarily burns fat for energy rather than carbohydrates. Here's a comprehensive explanation of the keto diet:*

### 1. Macronutrient Ratios:
*The keto diet is characterized by specific macronutrient ratios:*

**High Fat:.** *Approximately 70-80% of daily calories come from fats.*

**Low Carbohydrates:** *Restricting carbs to around 5-10% of daily calories.*

**Moderate Protein:** *Protein intake is moderate, around 10-20% of daily calories.*

### 2. Ketosis:
*The core principle of the keto diet is to induce and maintain a state of ketosis. When carbohydrate intake is*

severely restricted, the body's primary source of energy shifts from glucose (sugar) to ketones (produced from fat).

This metabolic shift encourages the body to use stored fat for fuel, resulting in weight loss.

### 3. Health Benefits:

The keto diet has been associated with several potential health benefits, including:

Weight Loss: Rapid fat burning can lead to weight loss, making it popular for those seeking to shed pounds.

**Improved Blood Sugar Control:** Ketosis can help stabilize blood sugar levels, making it an option for some people with diabetes.

**Enhanced Mental Clarity:** Some individuals report increased mental focus and clarity.

**Potential Treatment for Epilepsy:** The keto diet has been used as a therapeutic option for certain epilepsy patients.

**Appetite Control:** High-fat foods can promote feelings of fullness, reducing overall calorie intake.

**Potential for Seizure Reduction:** The keto diet may reduce the frequency and severity of seizures in some individuals with epilepsy.

### 4. Foods to Emphasize:

On the keto diet, you should emphasize:

Healthy Fats: Sources include avocados, olive oil, coconut oil, and nuts.

*Low-Carb Vegetables: Leafy greens, broccoli, cauliflower, and other non-starchy veggies.*
  *Moderate Protein: Lean meats, fish, and poultry.*
  *Dairy: Full-fat dairy products like cheese and yogurt (in moderation).*
   *Eggs: A rich source of fat and protein.*
  *Nuts and Seeds: Almonds, chia seeds, and walnuts are good choices.*
  ***Berries:*** *Some low-carb fruits like berries can be consumed in moderation.*

### 5. Foods to Avoid:

*Carbohydrate-rich foods and sugary items are restricted on the keto diet, including bread, pasta, rice, sugary snacks, and most fruits.*

### 6. Challenges and Considerations:

*The keto diet can be challenging to maintain, and it may not be suitable for everyone. Some considerations include:*
  ***Nutrient Deficiency:*** *A strict keto diet can lead to nutrient deficiencies if not carefully planned.*
   ***Potential Side Effects:*** *Some people experience the "keto flu," which includes symptoms like fatigue, headache, and irritability.*
  ***Limited Food Choices:*** *The diet may feel restrictive due to the elimination of many common foods.*
  ***Difficulty Sustaining:*** *Some individuals find it challenging to maintain the keto diet in the long term.*

### 7. Consult a Healthcare Provider:

*If you're considering the keto diet, it's essential to consult a healthcare provider or registered dietitian to ensure it's safe and appropriate for your individual health goals and needs.*

*The keto diet is a low-carb, high-fat eating plan designed to induce ketosis, which can lead to weight loss and other potential health benefits. It's a specialized diet that may work for some individuals, but it's important to consult with a healthcare provider or dietitian to determine if it's a suitable and safe option for you.*

# CHAPTER 25

## The Vegan Diet: A Plant-Powered Lifestyle.

*A vegan diet is a plant-based eating pattern that excludes all animal products, including meat, dairy, eggs, and even non-food animal-derived products like honey and gelatin. Here's a comprehensive explanation of the vegan diet:*

### 1. Plant-Based Focus:

*A vegan diet centers on plant foods, including fruits, vegetables, grains, legumes, nuts, seeds, and plant-based alternatives to animal products.*

### 2. Exclusion of Animal Products:

*Vegans avoid all animal-derived products, including:*

*__Meat:__  This includes beef, poultry, pork, and other animal meats.*

*__Dairy:__  No milk, cheese, yogurt, or butter from cows or other animals.*

*__Eggs:__  All types of eggs are excluded.*

*__Honey:__ Because it's produced by bees, it's not considered vegan.*

*__Gelatin:__  A common animal-derived ingredient in many processed foods and supplements.*

**Animal-Based Additives:** *Vegans avoid any food additives derived from animals.*

### 3. Nutrient Considerations:

*A vegan diet can be nutritious, but it may require attention to certain nutrients:*

**Protein:** *Plant-based protein sources include legumes, tofu, tempeh, and seitan.*

**Calcium:** *Fortified plant-based milk, tofu, leafy greens, and almonds are good sources.*

**Vitamin B12:** *This essential nutrient is often obtained through fortified foods or supplements.*

**Iron:** *Sources include beans, lentils, tofu, and fortified cereals.*

**Omega-3 Fatty Acids:** *Flaxseeds, chia seeds, and walnuts are sources of ALA, a type of omega-3. Vegans may consider algae-based supplements for DHA and EPA omega-3s.*

**Vitamin D:** *Exposure to sunlight and fortified foods are common sources.*

**Iodine:** *Iodized salt and some seaweed can provide iodine.*

**Zinc:** *Legumes, nuts, seeds, and whole grains contain zinc.*

### 4. Health Benefits:

*A well-balanced vegan diet offers several potential health benefits, including:*

**Lower Risk of Chronic Diseases:** *Reduced risk of heart disease, type 2 diabetes, and some cancers.*

**Weight Management:** *Many people find it easier to manage their weight on a vegan diet.*
**Improved Digestion:** *High fiber intake supports healthy digestion.*
**Ethical and Environmental Benefits:** *Veganism aligns with ethical concerns about animal welfare and environmental sustainability.*

## 5. Ethical and Environmental Aspects:

*Many people choose a vegan diet for ethical reasons, as it reduces harm to animals. Additionally, plant-based diets are often considered more environmentally sustainable due to reduced greenhouse gas emissions and land use.*

## 6. Challenges:

*Some challenges associated with a vegan diet include:*
**Meeting Nutritional Needs:** *Paying attention to certain nutrients like B12, iron, and calcium is essential.*
**Social Situations:** *Dining out or attending social events may require careful food choices.*
**Limited Convenience Options:** *Fast-food and pre-packaged meal options may be limited.*

## 7. Plant-Based Alternatives:

*The growing popularity of veganism has led to a wide range of plant-based alternatives to traditional animal products, including plant-based milks, cheeses, and meat substitutes.*

## 8. Ethical Considerations:

*Beyond health and the environment, veganism is often motivated by ethical concerns related to animal welfare and the treatment of animals in the food industry.*

*The vegan diet is a plant-powered lifestyle that excludes all animal products. It offers numerous health and ethical benefits but requires attention to certain nutrients to ensure nutritional adequacy. Consulting with a registered dietitian can provide guidance on how to thrive on a vegan diet while meeting your individual health and dietary needs.*

# CHAPTER 26

## The Paleo Diet: Eating Like Our Ancestors:

*The paleo diet, short for Paleolithic diet, is a dietary regimen inspired by the presumed eating habits of our distant ancestors during the Paleolithic era, a period around 2.5 million to 10,000 years ago. The core idea behind the paleo diet is to emulate the foods our hunter-gatherer ancestors would have consumed. Here's a comprehensive explanation of the paleo diet:*

### 1. Emphasis on Whole Foods:

*The paleo diet prioritizes whole, unprocessed foods, including:*

*__Lean Meats:__ Such as beef, poultry, and game meats.*
*__Fish:__ Especially fatty fish like salmon.*
*__Eggs:__ Ideally from pastured or free-range chickens.*
*__Vegetables:__ A wide variety of non-starchy vegetables.*
*__Fruits:__ Limited due to sugar content but still included.*
*__Nuts and Seeds:__ Almonds, walnuts, and others are encouraged.*
*__Healthy Fats:__ From sources like avocados, coconut oil, and olive oil.*

### 2. Exclusion of Processed Foods:

*Highly processed foods, refined sugars, grains, legumes, dairy products, and artificial additives are largely avoided.*

### 3. Dairy and Grains:

*Dairy products, such as milk, cheese, and yogurt, are excluded. Grains, including wheat, rice, and corn, are not part of the paleo diet due to their relatively recent introduction to human diets.*

### 4. Legumes:

*Legumes like beans, lentils, and peanuts are typically avoided because they contain anti-nutrients and phytates.*

### 5. Focus on Protein:

*Protein is a central component of the paleo diet. Lean meats and fish provide high-quality protein while aiding in satiety.*

### 6. Benefits:

*Advocates of the paleo diet claim several potential benefits, including:*

***Weight Loss:*** *Reducing processed and high-calorie foods can support weight management.*

***Improved Blood Sugar Control:*** *Limiting sugar and processed carbs may stabilize blood sugar levels.*

***Better Digestion:*** *Emphasizing whole foods can promote healthy digestion.*

**Allergy Management:** *Avoiding common allergens like wheat and dairy may benefit individuals with sensitivities.*

### 7. Challenges:

*Challenges associated with the paleo diet include:*

**Nutritional Balance:** *Some nutrients found in grains, legumes, and dairy products may need to be sourced from alternative foods.*

**Sustainability:** *Critics argue that the paleo diet's emphasis on meat may not be environmentally sustainable.*

**Limited Food Choices:** *The diet can feel restrictive to some individuals, particularly those accustomed to a more diverse diet.*

### 8. Evolutionary Perspective:

*The paleo diet is founded on the premise that our genes have evolved over thousands of years to thrive on the foods our ancestors consumed. Advocates argue that modern dietary changes have outpaced our genetic adaptation.*

### 9. Customization:

*There's room for customization within the paleo diet, allowing individuals to tailor it to their preferences and nutritional needs.*

### 10. Consultation:

*As with any diet, it's a good idea to consult with a healthcare provider or registered dietitian before embarking on a significant dietary change like the paleo diet to ensure it aligns with your health goals and needs.*

*The paleo diet is based on the concept of eating like our Paleolithic ancestors. While it emphasizes whole, unprocessed foods, it may not be suitable for everyone, and its long-term health effects are a subject of ongoing debate. Consulting with a healthcare provider or registered dietitian can offer guidance on whether the paleo diet is a good fit for your dietary goals.*

# CHAPTER 27

## Special Dietary Considerations: Catering to Unique Nutritional Needs:

*Special dietary considerations refer to dietary patterns tailored to meet the unique nutritional needs and requirements of specific individuals due to health conditions, allergies, ethical beliefs, or lifestyle choices. These considerations play a vital role in promoting individual health and well-being. Here's a comprehensive explanation of special dietary considerations:*

### 1. Medical Conditions:

*Many individuals have specific medical conditions that necessitate special dietary considerations:*

**Diabetes:** *People with diabetes must manage their carbohydrate intake and monitor blood sugar levels.*

**Celiac Disease:** *Those with celiac disease must avoid gluten-containing foods.*

**Food Allergies:** *Allergies to common foods like nuts, dairy, or shellfish require strict avoidance.*

**Heart Disease:** *A heart-healthy diet may be recommended to manage cholesterol and blood pressure.*

**Kidney Disease:** Reduced sodium and protein intake is often necessary.

**Gastrointestinal Disorders:** Conditions like irritable bowel syndrome (IBS) may require a low-FODMAP diet.

**Inflammatory Conditions:** Anti-inflammatory diets can be beneficial for conditions like rheumatoid arthritis.

**Cancer:** Some cancer patients require modified diets to manage side effects of treatment.

### 2. Allergies and Intolerances:

Food allergies and intolerances necessitate the avoidance of specific foods or ingredients. Common examples include gluten intolerance, lactose intolerance, and shellfish allergies.

### 3. Vegan and Vegetarian Diets:

Some individuals choose vegan or vegetarian diets for ethical, environmental, or health reasons. These diets require careful planning to ensure adequate nutrient intake.

### 4. Ethical and Environmental Concerns:

People who follow diets such as vegetarianism or veganism are often motivated by ethical concerns related to animal welfare and environmental sustainability.

### 5. Lifestyle Choices:

*Some people adopt dietary patterns based on lifestyle choices, such as low-carb diets, intermittent fasting, or specific meal timing strategies.*

### 6. Cultural and Religious Practices:

*Cultural and religious dietary practices are often influenced by traditions and observances. These diets can vary widely and may involve specific fasting periods or dietary restrictions.*

### 7. Weight Management:

*Many individuals choose dietary patterns focused on weight management and body composition goals. These include calorie counting, portion control, and macronutrient manipulation.*

### 8. Sustainability and Environmental Concerns:

*Sustainable diets prioritize foods with lower environmental impacts. They often include plant-based foods and minimize animal products.*

### 9. Individualized Nutrition:

*Special dietary considerations underscore the importance of individualized nutrition. What works for one person may not be suitable for another, and personalized dietary approaches are increasingly recognized as critical for optimizing health.*

### 10. Consultation:

*For anyone with unique dietary needs or questions, consultation with a healthcare provider, registered* dietitian, or nutrition specialist is highly recommended. These professionals can provide guidance, create personalized dietary plans, and monitor progress to ensure that dietary goals are met safely and effectively.

Special dietary considerations are essential for promoting health and well-being among individuals with specific needs or preferences. Whether driven by medical conditions, ethical beliefs, cultural practices, or lifestyle choices, these dietary patterns are integral to the diverse and individualized world of nutrition. Consulting with a qualified professional is often the first step in addressing and managing special dietary requirements.

# CHAPTER 28

## Sugar and Its Impact on Health: A Sweet but Complex Story

*Sugar is a type of carbohydrate found naturally in many foods and added to others for flavor. While it provides sweetness and energy, excessive sugar consumption has been associated with various health concerns. Here's a comprehensive explanation of sugar and its impact on health:*

### 1. Types of Sugar:
*There are two main types of sugar:*
***Natural Sugars:*** *Found in foods like fruits, vegetables, and milk. These sugars are accompanied by fiber, vitamins, and minerals.*
***Added Sugars:*** *Sugars added to foods and beverages during processing or preparation. Common sources include sugar-sweetened beverages, candies, and baked goods.*

### 2. Sugar and Energy:
*Sugar is a source of energy for the body. When consumed, it's broken down into glucose, which provides fuel for cells and bodily functions.*

### 3. Health Impact of Excessive Sugar Intake:

Overconsumption of added sugars has been linked to several health concerns:

**Obesity:** High sugar intake, especially from sugary beverages, can contribute to weight gain and obesity.

**Type 2 Diabetes:** Excessive sugar consumption may increase the risk of developing type 2 diabetes by influencing insulin resistance.

**Heart Health:.** High sugar intake can elevate triglycerides and increase the risk of heart disease.

**Dental Health:** Sugar is a primary contributor to tooth decay and cavities, especially when consumed in sugary foods and beverages.

**Fatty Liver Disease:** Excessive sugar intake, particularly fructose, may contribute to non-alcoholic fatty liver disease.

**Inflammation:** High sugar diets can promote inflammation in the body, which is associated with chronic diseases.

**Mood and Mental Health:** Sugar intake may affect mood, with some individuals experiencing sugar "crashes" and mood swings.

### 4. Hidden Sugars:

Added sugars can be "hidden" in processed foods under various names like high-fructose corn syrup, sucrose, and maltose. Reading food labels is essential to identify these sources.

### 5. Sugar Recommendations:

*Health organizations, including the World Health Organization (WHO) and the American Heart Association (AHA), provide guidelines for sugar intake. These organizations recommend limiting added sugar intake to no more than 10% of daily calories.*

### 6. Natural vs. Added Sugars:

*The sugars found in whole foods like fruits and vegetables come with essential nutrients and fiber, which can help slow sugar absorption and minimize its impact on blood sugar levels. In contrast, added sugars in processed foods lack these benefits.*

### 7. Moderation and Balance:

*Consuming sugar in moderation and as part of a balanced diet is key. It's possible to enjoy sweet treats and sugary foods occasionally without detrimental effects.*

### 8. Reducing Sugar Intake:

**Reducing sugar consumption can be achieved by:**

*Choosing whole foods over processed ones.*

*Opting for unsweetened or minimally processed foods.*

*Limiting sugary beverages*

*Reading food labels and being aware of added sugar content.*

### 9. Individual Variability:

*Individual responses to sugar can vary. Some people may be more sensitive to its effects, while others can tolerate it in larger amounts.*

### 10. Consultation:

*For personalized dietary guidance, individuals with specific health concerns related to sugar intake should consult with a healthcare provider or registered dietitian.*

*Sugar can be part of a balanced diet when consumed in moderation, primarily from natural sources like fruits and vegetables. However, excessive consumption of added sugars is associated with several health concerns, highlighting the importance of reading food labels and being mindful of sugar intake to support overall health and well-being.*

# CHAPTER 29

## Salt and Sodium: Roles and Risks in Health

*Salt and sodium are essential components in the human diet, playing crucial roles in various bodily functions. However, excessive sodium intake can lead to health risks. Here's a comprehensive explanation of salt and sodium, their roles, and potential health risks:*

### 1. Sodium in Salt:

*Salt, chemically known as sodium chloride (NaCl), is composed of sodium and chloride ions. Sodium is the component of salt that has the most significant impact on health.*

### 2. Role of Sodium:

*Sodium serves several essential functions in the body, including:*

***Fluid Balance:*** *Sodium helps maintain the balance of fluids in and around cells, tissues, and organs.*

***Nerve Function:*** *It plays a vital role in nerve transmission and communication between nerve cells.*

***Muscle Function:*** *Sodium is necessary for muscle contraction, including the heartbeat.*

**Blood Pressure Regulation:** *Sodium levels in the blood affect blood pressure.*

### 3. Dietary Sources of Sodium:

*Sodium is found naturally in many foods, especially fruits and vegetables, and is often added to foods during processing. Major sources of dietary sodium include:*

**Table salt.**

*Processed and pre-packaged foods, including canned soups, snacks, and processed meats.*

*Restaurant and fast-food items.*

*Baking soda and baking powder.*

### 4. Health Risks of Excessive Sodium Intake:

*While sodium is essential, excessive consumption can lead to health risks:*

**High Blood Pressure:** *High sodium intake is associated with elevated blood pressure, a significant risk factor for heart disease and stroke.*

**Heart Disease:** *High blood pressure, in turn, is a leading risk factor for heart disease.*

**Stroke:** *Elevated blood pressure contributes to an increased risk of stroke.*

**Kidney Disease:** *Excessive sodium intake can strain the kidneys, potentially leading to kidney disease.*

**Osteoporosis:** *Some research suggests that high sodium intake may be associated with bone loss, which can contribute to osteoporosis.*

### 5. Dietary Guidelines for Sodium:

Health organizations like the World Health Organization (WHO) and the American Heart Association (AHA) provide guidelines for sodium intake. They recommend limiting sodium intake to less than 2,300 milligrams (about 1 teaspoon of salt) per day.

### 6. Reducing Sodium Intake:
To reduce sodium intake, consider the following strategies:
Choose fresh, whole foods over processed and pre-packaged items.
Cook at home and use herbs and spices to season food instead of salt.
Read food labels to identify high-sodium products.
Limit the consumption of restaurant and fast-food meals.

### 7. Individual Variability:
People's sensitivity to sodium can vary. Some individuals may be more prone to the blood pressure-raising effects of sodium.

### 8. Hydration Balance:
Sodium is intricately linked with fluid balance in the body. Maintaining a proper balance of sodium and water is essential for overall health.

### 9. Consultation:
For personalized dietary guidance or individuals with specific health concerns related to sodium intake, it's

*advisable to consult with a healthcare provider or registered dietitian.*

*Salt and sodium are essential for various bodily functions, but excessive sodium intake can lead to health risks, particularly high blood pressure and related conditions. Being mindful of sodium consumption and following dietary guidelines can support overall health and well-being.*

# CHAPTER 30

## Fiber: The Digestive Health Hero

*Fiber is a dietary component found in plant-based foods that plays a vital role in promoting digestive health and overall well-being. It offers numerous benefits that go beyond just regularity. Here's a comprehensive explanation of fiber and its role in digestive health:*

### 1. Types of Fiber:
*There are two main types of dietary fiber:*
**Soluble Fiber:** *Dissolves in water and forms a gel-like substance in the digestive tract. Found in foods like oats, beans, and fruits.*
**Insoluble Fiber:** *Does not dissolve in water and adds bulk to stool, aiding in bowel movements. Common sources include whole grains, vegetables, and bran.*

### 2. Digestive Health Benefits:
*Fiber offers several digestive health benefits:*
**Regular Bowel Movements:** *Insoluble fiber adds bulk to stool, preventing constipation and promoting regular bowel movements.*
**Prevention of Diarrhea:** *Soluble fiber can help absorb excess water in the intestines, preventing diarrhea.*

**Diverticulitis Prevention:** A high-fiber diet may reduce the risk of diverticulitis, a condition characterized by inflammation or infection of small pouches in the colon.

**Hemorrhoid Prevention:** Fiber helps prevent hemorrhoids by promoting soft, bulky stools that are easy to pass.

**Gut Microbiome Health:** Fiber serves as a food source for beneficial gut bacteria, supporting a healthy gut microbiome.

**Colon Health:** A diet rich in fiber may reduce the risk of colon cancer.

### 3. Weight Management:

Fiber promotes feelings of fullness and satiety, which can aid in weight management by reducing overall calorie intake.

### 4. Blood Sugar Control:

Soluble fiber can help stabilize blood sugar levels by slowing the absorption of sugar from the digestive tract.

### 5. Heart Health:

High-fiber diets are associated with reduced risk factors for heart disease, including lower cholesterol levels and blood pressure.

### 6. Food Sources of Fiber:

Fiber is abundant in plant-based foods, including:
Whole grains: Brown rice, whole wheat, oats.

**Fruits:** Apples, pears, berries.

*Vegetables: Broccoli, carrots, spinach.*
*Legumes: Beans, lentils, chickpeas.*
*Nuts and seeds: Almonds, chia seeds, flaxseeds.*

### 7. Daily Fiber Intake:
*Health organizations recommended daily fiber intake of 25 to 38 grams for adults, depending on age and gender. However, most people fall short of meeting these recommendations.*

### 8. Gradual Increase:
*It's advisable to increase fiber intake gradually to prevent digestive discomfort, such as bloating and gas.*

### 9. Hydration:
*Consuming enough water is essential when increasing fiber intake to aid in the passage of fiber through the digestive system.*

### 10. Consultation:
*For individuals with specific dietary concerns or health conditions, it's beneficial to consult with a healthcare provider or registered dietitian for personalized dietary guidance.*

*Fiber is an essential component of a healthy diet and a digestive health hero. Incorporating a variety of fiber-rich foods into your meals can support regularity, prevent digestive issues, and provide a range of health benefits. It's an important dietary element that contributes to overall well-being.*

# CHAPTER 31

## Water: The Forgotten Nutrient

*Water is often referred to as the "forgotten nutrient" because it doesn't receive as much attention as other nutrients like protein, carbohydrates, and vitamins. Yet, water is arguably the most vital nutrient for our survival and well-being. Here's a comprehensive explanation of water and its crucial role in our health:*

### 1. The Importance of Water:
*Water is essential for life and is involved in nearly every bodily function. It makes up a significant portion of our body weight, and without an adequate supply of water, we cannot survive.*

### 2. Roles of Water:
*Water plays several critical roles in the body:*
***Hydration:*** *It's vital for maintaining the balance of bodily fluids and preventing dehydration.*
***Temperature Regulation:*** *Water helps regulate body temperature by releasing heat through perspiration.*
***Digestion and Nutrient Absorption:***

Water is needed for the breakdown of food and the absorption of nutrients in the digestive system.

 **Transport of Nutrients and Oxygen:** Blood, composed mostly of water, carries nutrients, oxygen, and waste products to and from cells.

 **Joint Lubrication:** Water helps lubricate joints, enabling smooth movement.

**Waste Removal:** Water assists in the removal of waste products from the body, primarily through urine.

**Brain and Nervous System Function:** Proper hydration is crucial for cognitive function and nerve transmission.

### 3. Daily Water Needs:

Daily water requirements vary depending on factors like age, activity level, climate, and individual health. A common guideline is the "8x8 rule," which suggests drinking eight 8-ounce glasses of water a day, totaling about 2 liters or half a gallon. However, individual needs may differ.

### 4. Thirst as a Signal:

Thirst is the body's way of signaling that it needs more water. It's essential to listen to your body and drink when you're thirsty.

### 5. Hydration from Foods:

Water can also be obtained from foods, particularly fruits and vegetables, which have high water content. This contributes to overall hydration.

### 6. Dehydration:

Dehydration occurs when the body loses more fluids than it takes in. It can lead to symptoms such as dry mouth, dark urine, fatigue, and dizziness. Severe dehydration is a medical emergency.

### 7. Overhydration:

While dehydration is a concern, excessive water intake can lead to a condition called hyponatremia, where the balance of electrolytes in the body is disrupted.

### 8. Individual Variability:

Hydration needs can vary significantly from person to person. Factors like activity level, climate, and medical conditions affect water requirements.

### 9. Water and Health:

Proper hydration is essential for overall health. It can improve skin health, support weight management, aid in digestion, and enhance cognitive function.

### 10. Consultation:

For individuals with specific concerns related to hydration, such as athletes or those with medical conditions, consulting with a healthcare provider or registered dietitian can provide personalized guidance on fluid intake.

Water is often overlooked as a nutrient, but it is vital for life and well-being. Proper hydration is essential for maintaining bodily functions and overall health. Listening *to your body's signals, staying adequately hydrated, and understanding your individual needs are all crucial for making water a part of a healthy lifestyle.*

# CHAPTER 32

## Food Labels and Understanding Nutrition Facts

*Food labels provide valuable information about the nutritional content of packaged foods, helping consumers make informed choices about their diet. Understanding the information on food labels is essential for making healthy and informed decisions. Here's a comprehensive explanation of food labels and how to interpret nutrition facts:*

### 1. Nutrition Facts Panel:

*The Nutrition Facts panel is a standard section on food labels that provides essential information about the product's nutritional content. It typically includes:*
*Serving Size:*
*The suggested serving size for the product.Calories:*
*The number of calories in one serving Macronutrients:*
*Information about macronutrients, including:*
***Total Fat:*** *The total amount of fat per serving.*
***Saturated Fat:*** *The amount of saturated fat per serving*
***Trans Fat:*** *The amount of trans fat, if present.*
***Cholesterol:*** *The cholesterol content per serving.*

**Sodium:** *The amount of sodium per serving.*
**Total Carbohydrates:** *The total carbs per serving.*
**Dietary Fiber:** *The amount of dietary fiber per serving*
**Sugars:** *The quantity of sugars per serving.*
**Protein:** *The protein content per serving.*

## 2. Percent Daily Value (%DV):

*The %DV indicates how much a nutrient in one serving of the food contributes to your daily diet based on a daily intake of 2,000 calories. It helps you assess whether a food is high or low in a specific nutrient.*

## 3. Ingredient List:

*The ingredient list details all the components in the product, with the main ingredients listed first. It can help you identify added sugars, preservatives, and other components you might want to avoid.*

## 4. Serving Size and Servings per Container:

*Pay attention to the serving size to ensure you're comparing like quantities when evaluating the nutritional information. The "servings per container" tells you how many servings are in the entire package.*

## 5. Daily Reference Values (DRVs):

*In addition to %DV, some labels may include Daily Reference Values for nutrients like fat, saturated fat, cholesterol, carbohydrates, dietary fiber, and sodium, based on a 2,000-calorie diet.*

## 6. Health Claims:

Some labels include health claims, such as "low in saturated fat" or "high in fiber." These claims are regulated by health authorities and can help you make healthier choices.

### 7. Nutrient Content Claims:

Nutrient content claims highlight specific attributes of the product, such as "low fat," "reduced sodium," or "high in vitamin C."

### 8. Be Mindful of Serving Sizes:

Pay attention to the serving size listed on the label. If you consume more or less than the specified serving, adjust the nutritional information accordingly.

### 9. Understand %DV:

A %DV of 5% or less is considered low, while 20% or more is high. Use %DV to quickly identify whether a food is a good or poor source of a specific nutrient.

### 10. Compare Products:

Use food labels to compare similar products and make choices that align with your dietary goals, whether you're aiming to reduce sodium intake, limit added sugars, or increase fiber consumption.

Understanding food labels empowers consumers to make informed choices about the foods they eat. It's a valuable tool for managing dietary preferences and nutritional goals. By learning how to interpret nutrition facts and ingredient lists, you can make healthier and *more conscious decisions about the foods you purchase and consume.*

# CHAPTER 33

## Controlled Portion and Mindful Eating: Keys to Healthy Eating Habits:

*Controlled portion and mindful eating are two essential practices that can promote healthier eating habits and overall well-being. They focus on awareness and moderation, helping individuals make better food choices and maintain a balanced diet. Here's a comprehensive explanation of controlled portion and mindful eating:*

### 1. What is a Controlled Portion?
*Controlled portion eating involves managing the size of food servings to ensure they align with your dietary needs and goals.*

### 2. Benefits of Controlled Portion:
*Weight Management: Controlling portion sizes can prevent overeating and support weight management.*
***Caloric Awareness:** It helps you become more aware of your calorie intake, making it easier to maintain or lose weight.*

***Balanced Nutrition:*** *It encourages a well-rounded diet by ensuring you get a variety of nutrients.*

***Prevents Overconsumption:*** *It reduces the risk of excessive calorie intake, which can lead to weight gain and related health issues.*

***Cost Savings:*** *Smaller portions can lead to less food waste and reduced grocery bills.*

### 3. Tips for Controlled Portion:

*Use measuring cups or a food scale to accurately determine serving sizes.*

*Eat from smaller plates to visually control portion sizes.*

*Practice mindful eating to savor each bite and recognize when you're satisfied.*

*Be mindful of restaurant serving sizes, which are often larger than needed.*

*Pre-portion snacks into smaller containers to avoid overindulging.*

### 4. What is Mindful Eating?

*Mindful eating is a practice that involves paying full attention to the sensory experience of eating, including the taste, texture, and aroma of food, as well as your body's hunger and fullness cues.*

### 5. Benefits of Mindful Eating:

***Improved Satisfaction:*** *Mindful eating can enhance your enjoyment of food by savoring each bite.*

***Better Digestion:*** *Eating slowly and mindfully can aid digestion.*

**Weight Management:** *It can help control emotional and binge eating, leading to weight maintenance.*

**Increased Awareness:** *Mindful eating encourages a greater awareness of body signals related to hunger and fullness.*

**Enhanced Food Choices:** *It helps you make healthier food choices and reduce impulsive or emotional eating.*

### 6. Tips for Mindful Eating:

*Eat without distractions, such as TV or smartphones.*

*Savor each bite and focus on the taste, texture, and smell of your food.*

*Listen to your body's hunger and fullness cues.*

*Eat slowly and chew your food thoroughly. Be aware of emotional eating triggers and address them in non-food ways.*

### 7. Combining Controlled Portion and Mindful Eating:

*Combining controlled portion eating with mindful eating can help you manage your food intake, enjoy your meals, and maintain a balanced diet. It encourages a more conscious and healthy relationship with food.*

*Controlled portions and mindful eating practices can contribute to healthier eating habits and support your overall well-being. By being mindful of portion sizes, listening to your body's cues, and savoring each bite, you can make more nutritious food choices, prevent overeating, and enjoy a positive relationship with food.*

# CHAPTER 34

## Food Allergies and Intolerances: Understanding the Differences

*Food allergies and food intolerances are two distinct but often confused conditions that involve adverse reactions to specific foods. Understanding the differences between them is essential for proper diagnosis, management, and dietary choices. Here's a comprehensive explanation of food allergies and intolerances.*

### 1. What is a Food Allergy?
*A food allergy is an abnormal immune response to a particular food protein. When someone with a food allergy consumes the allergenic food, their immune system identifies it as a threat and produces an allergic reaction.*

### 2. Common Food Allergens:
*Common food allergens include peanuts, tree nuts, eggs, milk, soy, wheat, fish, and shellfish.*

### 3. Symptoms of Food Allergies:

Symptoms can range from mild to severe and may include:
Skin reactions (hives, itching, swelling).
Gastrointestinal issues (nausea, vomiting, diarrhea).
Respiratory symptoms (wheezing, coughing, shortness of breath).
Anaphylaxis: A severe, life-threatening reaction involving swelling of the throat, a drop in blood pressure, and difficulty breathing.

## 4. Diagnosis and Management:

Food allergies are typically diagnosed through allergy testing, which may include skin prick tests or blood tests. The primary management strategy is strict avoidance of the allergenic food.

## 5. What is Food Intolerance?

Food intolerance, unlike allergies, doesn't involve the immune system. It occurs when the body has difficulty digesting or processing a specific component of food. The most common intolerances are to lactose (milk sugar), fructose (fruit sugar), and gluten.

## 6. Common Food Intolerances:

Common food intolerances include lactose intolerance (inability to digest lactose), fructose malabsorption (difficulty digesting fructose), and non-celiac gluten sensitivity (sensitivity to gluten without having celiac disease).

## 7. Symptoms of Food Intolerances:

*Symptoms can vary widely and may include:*
*Gastrointestinal symptoms (bloating, gas, diarrhea, stomach cramps).*
*Headaches or migraines.*
*Skin issues (rashes, eczema).*
*Fatigue.*

### 8. Diagnosis and Management:

*Food intolerances are typically diagnosed through a combination of symptom assessment and dietary exclusion trials. Management often involves reducing or eliminating the offending component from the diet, but total avoidance of the food is not required.*

### Key Differences:

**Immune Response:** *Allergies involve the immune system's response, while intolerances do not.*
**Severity:** *Allergies can be life-threatening, while intolerances are generally less severe.*
**Diagnosis:** *Allergies are diagnosed through allergy tests, while intolerances are often identified through symptom evaluation and dietary trials.*
**Management:** *Allergies require strict avoidance, whereas intolerances may allow some tolerance of the food.*

*Understanding the differences between food allergies and intolerances is essential for proper diagnosis and management. If you suspect you have a food allergy or intolerance, consult with a healthcare provider or allergist for accurate testing and guidance on dietary modifications.*

# CHAPTER 35

## Nutritional Myths and Facts: Separating Fiction from Reality

*Nutrition is a field often filled with myths and misconceptions. It's crucial to differentiate between fact and fiction to make informed dietary choices. Here are some common nutritional myths, along with the corresponding facts:*

***Myth 1:*** *Carbohydrates Make You Gain Weight.*
***Fact:*** *Carbohydrates are a fundamental source of energy and are not inherently fattening. Weight gain typically occurs when you consume excess calories, regardless of the nutrient source. Choosing complex carbohydrates like whole grains, fruits, and vegetables can be part of a healthy diet.*

***Myth 2:*** *All Fats Are Unhealthy.*
***Fact:*** *Not all fats are created equal. While trans fats and excessive saturated fats can be harmful, healthy fats like those found in avocados, nuts, and fatty fish are essential for overall health. They support brain function, hormone production, and the absorption of fat-soluble vitamins.*

***Myth 3:*** *Skipping Meals Helps with Weight Loss.*
   ***Fact:*** *Skipping meals can lead to overeating later in the day and can negatively impact metabolism. Regular, balanced meals and snacks can support weight management and provide consistent energy.*

***Myth 4:*** *You Need to Detox Your Body.*
   ***Fact:*** *The body has its detoxification mechanisms, primarily involving the liver and kidneys. Detox diets or products are generally unnecessary and may be harmful. A balanced diet with plenty of water supports natural detoxification.*

***Myth 5:*** *Eating Late at Night Causes Weight Gain.*
   *Fact: Weight gain is related to overall calorie intake and expenditure, not the timing of meals. If late-night eating leads to excessive calorie consumption, it can contribute to weight gain, but the time itself is not the primary factor.*

***Myth 6:*** *Gluten-Free Diets Are Healthier for Everyone.*
   ***Fact:*** *Gluten-free diets are essential for those with celiac disease or gluten sensitivity, but they are not inherently healthier for individuals without these conditions. Many gluten-free products are less nutritious and may lack essential nutrients.*

***Myth 7:*** *Organic Foods Are Always Healthier.*
   ***Fact:*** *Organic foods are grown without synthetic pesticides, but they are not necessarily more nutritious.*

*The choice between organic and conventional foods depends on factors like personal preference and environmental concerns.*

**Myth 8:** *Eating Egg Yolks Is Unhealthy Due to Cholesterol.*
  **Fact:** *Recent research indicates that dietary cholesterol, like that in egg yolks, has a minimal impact on blood cholesterol levels for most people. Eggs are nutrient-rich and can be part of a healthy diet.*

**Myth 9:** *Supplements Can Replace a Balanced Diet.*
  **Fact:** *While supplements can be beneficial for certain nutrient deficiencies, they are not a substitute for a well-rounded diet. Whole foods provide a wide range of nutrients, fiber, and phytochemicals that supplements cannot replicate.*

**Myth 10:** *You Should Avoid All Sugar.*
  **Fact:** *While excessive added sugars are linked to health issues, you don't need to eliminate all sugars from your diet. Naturally occurring sugars in fruits and dairy products come with essential nutrients and are a healthier choice than added sugars in processed foods.*

*Understanding these nutritional myths and facts can help you make more informed dietary choices. For personalized guidance on your nutrition, consult with a registered dietitian or healthcare professional.*

# CHAPTER 36

## Cooking and Food Preparation Techniques: Enhancing Your Culinary Skills

*Mastering cooking and food preparation techniques can elevate your culinary skills, making home-cooked meals more delicious and enjoyable. Here are various techniques and tips to enhance your skills in the kitchen:*

### 1. Knife Skills:

*Proper knife techniques, including chopping, dicing, and slicing, can make food preparation more efficient and safer. Invest in a good-quality chef's knife and practice your knife skills regularly.*

### 2. Mise en Place:

*This French term means "everything in its place." It involves preparing and organizing all ingredients before cooking. Mise en place helps streamline the cooking process and ensures you have everything you need.*

### 3. Sauteing and Stir-Frying:

*Mastering the art of sautéing and stir-frying allows you to quickly cook vegetables, meats, and other ingredients* while retaining their texture and flavor. Use high heat and keep ingredients moving in the pan.

### 4. Roasting and Baking:

Roasting and baking are dry-heat cooking methods that create delicious, caramelized flavors. They're perfect for dishes like roasted vegetables, chicken, and baked goods.

### 5. Grilling:

Grilling adds smoky, charred flavors to foods. Whether you're grilling vegetables, meats, or seafood, understanding heat zones and proper timing is key.

### 6. Braising and Stewing:

These slow-cooking techniques involve simmering ingredients in liquid, resulting in tender and flavorful dishes. Perfect for dishes like pot roast and stews.

### 7. Poaching:

Poaching involves gently simmering ingredients in liquid, typically water or broth. It's a delicate method used for cooking items like eggs, fish, and chicken.

### 8. Steaming:

Steaming is a healthy way to cook food while retaining its natural flavors and nutrients. It's ideal for vegetables, seafood, and dumplings.

### 9. Blanching and Shocking:

Blanching involves briefly boiling vegetables before quickly cooling them in ice water. This preserves their color and texture and is often used in salads.

### 10. Emulsification:

Emulsification is the process of combining two liquids that don't naturally mix, like oil and vinegar, to create stable mixtures like vinaigrettes and mayonnaise.

### 11. Reduction:

Reducing liquids, such as wine or broth, intensifies flavors and creates sauces or glazes. It's a technique used in making pan sauces and gravies.

### 12. Seasoning:

Proper seasoning with salt, pepper, herbs, and spices enhances the flavor of your dishes. Taste and adjust seasoning as you cook.

### 13. Plating and Presentation:

How you present a dish can significantly affect the dining experience. Experiment with different plating techniques and garnishes to make your meals visually appealing.

### 14. Food Safety:

Understanding food safety practices, including proper food storage, handling, and cooking temperatures, is crucial to prevent foodborne illnesses.

### 15. Recipe Adaptation:

*Don't be afraid to adapt recipes to suit your taste and dietary preferences. Learning when and how to substitute ingredients is a valuable skill.*

### 16. Culinary Basics:
*Master the fundamental techniques, such as creating a roux for sauces, making a vinaigrette, and understanding various cooking methods, to build a strong culinary foundation.*

### 17. Experimentation:
*Don't be afraid to try new ingredients and techniques. Experimentation is one of the best ways to learn and grow as a cook.*

### 18. Practice and Patience:
*Like any skill, cooking improves with practice and patience. Be prepared for some failures, but they are valuable learning experiences.*

*Enhancing your cooking and food preparation techniques can turn meal preparation into a rewarding and enjoyable experience. Whether you're a beginner or an experienced cook, continuous learning and experimentation in the kitchen can lead to delicious, restaurant-quality meals at home.*

# CHAPTER 37

## Eating Disorders and Their Effects

*Eating disorders are complex mental health conditions characterized by disturbances in eating behaviors and a preoccupation with body weight, shape, and size. They can have severe physical, emotional, and social effects. Here's an overview of common eating disorders and their effects:*

### 1. Anorexia Nervosa:

*Effects:  Anorexia is characterized by extreme food restriction, fear of gaining weight, and a distorted body image. Its effects can include:*
*Severe malnutrition and weight loss.*
*Weakened immune system.*
*Cardiac issues, including arrhythmias and heart failure.*
*Cognitive and emotional disturbances, such as anxiety, depression, and obsession with food and weight.*
*Social isolation and strained relationships.*

### 2. Bulimia Nervosa:

**Effects:** Bulimia involves cycles of binge eating followed by purging behaviors like vomiting, excessive exercise, or laxative use. Its effects can include:

Electrolyte imbalances, leading to cardiac issues.
Gastrointestinal problems.
Dental issues due to stomach acid exposure.
Emotional distress, including guilt and shame.
Weight fluctuations.
Social withdrawal and secrecy.

### 3. Binge-Eating Disorder:

**Effects:** Binge-eating disorder involves recurrent episodes of consuming large amounts of food without purging. Its effects can include:

Obesity and related health concerns.
Emotional distress and guilt.
Increased risk of heart disease and type 2 diabetes.
Low self-esteem and depression.
Social isolation.

### 4. Avoidant/Restrictive Food Intake Disorder (ARFID):

**Effects:** ARFID is characterized by limited food preferences and avoidance of certain foods or food groups. Its effects can include:

Nutritional deficiencies and failure to thrive (especially in children).
Impaired physical growth and development.
Limited social activities due to dietary restrictions.
Anxiety and stress related to mealtimes.

### 5. Other Specified Feeding or Eating Disorder (OSFED):

*Effects:* OSFED includes a range of disordered eating behaviors that do not meet the criteria for other specific eating disorders. Its effects vary based on the specific behaviors but can include physical and emotional consequences.

### 6. Effects on Mental Health:

Eating disorders often co-occur with other mental health conditions like depression, anxiety, and obsessive-compulsive disorder, compounding the emotional and psychological toll.

### 7. Social and Relationship Effects:

Eating disorders can lead to social isolation, strained relationships, and withdrawal from social activities due to the preoccupation with food, weight, and appearance.

### 8. Long-Term Health Consequences:

Untreated eating disorders can lead to severe, long-term health issues, including heart problems, bone loss, organ damage, and even death.

### 9. Recovery and Treatment:

Treatment for eating disorders typically involves a combination of medical, nutritional, and psychological therapies. Recovery is possible, but it often requires professional help, social support, and a long-term commitment to change.

*Eating disorders are serious conditions that can have profound effects on physical health, emotional well-being, and social functioning. Early recognition and intervention are crucial to prevent long-term consequences and promote recovery. If you or someone you know is struggling with an eating disorder, seeking help from a healthcare professional is essential.*

# CHAPTER 38

## Nutritional Supplements: Pros and Con

*Nutritional supplements, such as vitamins, minerals, and herbal products, are commonly used to complement a person's diet or address specific health concerns. While they can provide benefits, they also come with potential drawbacks. Here's an overview of the pros and cons of using nutritional supplements:*

**Pros:**

### 1. Nutrient Deficiency Prevention:
*Pro: Supplements can help fill nutrient gaps in your diet, preventing deficiencies, especially if you have dietary restrictions or specific health conditions.*

### 2. Convenience:
*Pro: Supplements offer a convenient way to ensure you get essential nutrients when whole foods are unavailable or inconvenient.*

### 3. Targeted Health Support:

*Pro:. Some supplements are designed to support specific health needs, such as bone health, heart health, or immune function.*

### 4. Athlete and Performance Enhancement:

*Pro: Athletes and active individuals may benefit from certain supplements that enhance performance, support muscle recovery, or improve endurance.*

### 5. Disease Management:

*Pro: Some supplements are used to manage specific medical conditions, such as folic acid for neural tube defects or vitamin D for osteoporosis.*

### 6. Antioxidant Protection:

*Pro: Antioxidant supplements like vitamin C and E can help protect the body from damage caused by free radicals and oxidative stress.*

### Cons:

### 1. Lack of Regulation:

*Con: The supplement industry is not as tightly regulated as the pharmaceutical industry, which means product safety and efficacy can vary widely.*

### 2. Overconsumption Risk:

*Con:. Excessive consumption of certain vitamins and minerals can lead to toxicities and adverse effects. It's essential to use supplements in moderation.*

### 3. Potential Interactions:

**Con:**  Some supplements can interact with medications or other supplements, leading to adverse effects or reduced effectiveness.

### 4. Cost:

**Con:**  High-quality supplements can be expensive, and relying on them to meet nutritional needs may strain your budget.

### 5. Food vs. Supplements:

**Con:** Whole foods offer a wide range of nutrients and other beneficial compounds that supplements cannot replicate. Relying on supplements alone may miss out on these benefits.

### 6. Uncertain Efficacy:

**Con:**  The effectiveness of many supplements is still under research. Some may not provide the expected health benefits or have limited scientific support.

### 7. Isolating Nutrients:

**Con:**  Taking individual nutrients in supplement form may not capture the synergistic effects of various compounds found in whole foods.

### 8. Risk of Misuse:

**Con:**  Some people may misuse supplements in an attempt to self-treat health conditions without proper guidance, potentially causing harm.

### 9. Not a Substitute for a Balanced Diet:

**Con:** *Supplements should complement a balanced diet but not replace it. Whole foods offer a wider range of nutrients, fiber, and health benefits.*

### 10. Quality Variability:

**Con:** *The quality and purity of supplements can vary widely among brands and products. Choosing reputable manufacturers is crucial.*

*In summary, nutritional supplements can be beneficial for addressing specific nutritional needs or health concerns, but they should be used thoughtfully. It's essential to consult with a healthcare professional before starting any new supplement regimen to ensure safety and effectiveness, and to avoid potential risks associated with misuse or overconsumption. Whole foods should remain the foundation of a healthy diet.*

# CHAPTER 39

## Meal Planning and Prepping: A Guide to Healthy Eating and Convenience

***Meal planning and prepping*** *are essential strategies for maintaining a healthy diet, saving time, and reducing food waste. Here's a guide to help you get started and make the most of these practices:*

***Meal Planning:***

### *1. Set Your Goals:*

*Determine your dietary goals, whether it's to eat healthier, save money, or lose weight. Your goals will influence your meal planning.*

### *2. Choose a Schedule:*

*Decide how often you want to plan meals, such as weekly or monthly. Weekly planning is common as it allows for flexibility.*

### *3. Create a Master List:*

*Start with a list of your favorite recipes, including breakfast, lunch, dinner, and snacks. You can reference this list when planning.*

### 4. Plan Your Meals:
*Decide which meals you'll prepare for the upcoming week or month. Consider variety, nutritional balance, and your schedule.*

### 5. Make a Grocery List:
*Create a shopping list based on the ingredients you need for your planned meals. This list reduces impulse purchases.*

### 6. Prepare in Advance:
*Choose a day for meal planning and grocery shopping. Having a set routine simplifies the process.*

### Meal Prepping:

### 7. Choose Your Prep Day:
*Dedicate a specific day for meal prep. Sunday is a popular choice, but any day that suits your schedule will work.*

### 8. Prepare Ingredients:
*Chop vegetables, portion proteins, and pre-cook grains and beans to have ingredients ready for your meals.*

### 9. Cook in Batches:

*Prepare larger quantities of food. For instance, make a big pot of soup, a tray of roasted vegetables, or a batch of rice.*

### 10. Portion Control:
*Use portion-sized containers to store individual meals. This makes it easy to grab a pre-portioned, balanced meal.*

### 11. Label and Date:
*Label containers with the date and contents to avoid confusion or food waste.*

### 12. Refrigerate or Freeze:
*Store meals in the refrigerator for short-term consumption or freeze them for longer-term use.*

### Benefits of Meal Planning and Prepping:

**1. Saves Time:** *You can prepare meals in advance, reducing the need for daily cooking.*

**2. Reduces Stress:** *Knowing what to eat each day eliminates mealtime stress and indecision.*

**3. Saves Money:** *Reduced dining out and fewer impulse grocery purchases can lead to cost savings.*

**4. Promotes Healthy Eating:** *Meal planning allows you to create balanced, nutritious meals.*

**5. Reduces Food Waste:** *Portioning meals and using ingredients efficiently minimizes food waste.*

**6. Supports Weight Management:** *Planned meals can help with portion control and calorie management.*

**7. Convenient Work and School Lunches:** *Prepped meals make it easy to pack lunches for work or school.*

**8. Enhances Variety:** *Meal planning helps you incorporate a wider range of foods into your diet.*

**Challenges:**

**1. Time Investment:** *Meal planning and prepping can require time upfront, but the time savings during the week often outweigh this.*

**2. Sticking to the Plan:** *Staying disciplined and following your meal plan can be challenging.*

**3. Lack of Variety:** *Repeating the same meals can become monotonous. Be sure to include variety in your planning.*

**4. Storage Space:** *Storing prepped meals in your refrigerator or freezer may require extra space.*

*Overall, meal planning and prepping are valuable strategies for achieving a healthy and convenient way of eating. They can help you make nutritious choices, save time, and reduce stress associated with mealtime decisions. With practice and flexibility, you can make these practices a regular part of your routine.*

# CHAPTER 40

## Dining Out Healthily: Tips for Making Smart Food Choices

*Eating out at restaurants or other food establishments doesn't mean you have to sacrifice your commitment to healthy eating. With some careful choices and strategies, you can enjoy dining out while still making nutritious decisions. Here are some tips for dining out healthily:*

### 1. Plan Ahead:

*Before heading to a restaurant, check out the menu online if possible. Look for healthier options and make a decision before you arrive.*

### 2. Choose the Right Restaurant:

*Opt for restaurants that offer a variety of menu items, including salads, lean proteins, and vegetable-based dishes. Avoid places with limited unhealthy options.*

### 3. Be Mindful of Portion Sizes:

*Restaurant portions are often larger than what you'd serve at home. Consider sharing a dish with a friend or asking for a to-go container right away to save half for later.*

### 4. Start with a Salad or Soup:
Having a salad or broth-based soup as an appetizer can help fill you up with fewer calories.

### 5. Select Lean Proteins:
Choose grilled, baked, or steamed options for proteins like chicken, fish, or tofu. Avoid fried or breaded items.

### 6. Watch the Sauces and Dressings:
Ask for sauces, dressings, and condiments on the side so you can control how much you use. Opt for vinaigrettes or tomato-based sauces over creamy or buttery ones.

### 7. Load Up on Veggies:
When possible, choose dishes with a variety of vegetables. Side dishes like steamed broccoli or mixed greens can be great additions.

### 8. Mind the Sides:
Opt for healthier side options like a side salad, steamed vegetables, or brown rice instead of fries or mashed potatoes.

### 9. Control Dessert:
If you want dessert, consider sharing it with others at your table. Alternatively, choose fruit, sorbet, or a smaller, lighter dessert.

### 10. Drink Wisely:

*Water, herbal tea, or a glass of wine can be better choices than sugary soft drinks or calorie-laden cocktails.*

### 11. Be Cautious with All-You-Can-Eat:
*Buffet-style or all-you-can-eat restaurants can be challenging. Focus on small portions and avoid overeating.*

### 12. Ask Questions:
*Don't hesitate to ask your server about the preparation of dishes or if substitutions are possible. They can often accommodate your preferences.*

### 13. Be Mindful of Hidden Calories:
*Watch for hidden sources of extra calories, like butter, cheese, or high-calorie toppings on salads and dishes.*

### 14. Practice Portion Control:
*If you can't share or save part of your meal, ask for a half portion or a takeout container right away.*

### 15. Listen to Your Body:
*Pay attention to your hunger and fullness cues. Eat slowly and savor your meal to avoid overeating.*

### 16. Treat Dining Out as an Occasional Splurge:
*While dining out healthily is possible, it's also okay to occasionally indulge in your favorite treats when you're at a restaurant. Balance is key.*

*Remember, dining out healthily is about making smart choices while still enjoying the experience. With these tips, you can savor restaurant meals without compromising your commitment to a nutritious diet.*

# CHAPTER 41

## Sustainable Eating and Ethical Food Choices: A Guide to Environmentally and Socially Responsible Eating

*Sustainable eating involves making food choices that are not only healthy for your body but also considerate of the environment and the welfare of animals and communities. Here are some guidelines to help you make ethical and sustainable food choices:*

### 1. Choose Local and Seasonal Produce:
*Opt for fruits and vegetables that are in season and grown locally. Supporting local farmers reduces the environmental impact of long-distance transportation and helps the local economy.*

### 2. Reduce Meat Consumption:
*Consider reducing your meat intake and incorporating more plant-based meals. Meat production has a significant environmental footprint, so choosing plant-based options can lower your carbon footprint.*

### 3. Support Sustainable Seafood:
Look for sustainably sourced seafood that is certified by organizations like the Marine Stewardship Council (MSC). These choices help protect our oceans and marine ecosystems.

### 4. Buy Organic and Non-GMO:
Choose organic and non-GMO (genetically modified organism) foods when possible. These options are typically grown with fewer pesticides and promote soil health.

### 5. Minimize Food Waste:
Plan your meals and use leftovers to reduce food waste. Composting can help divert food scraps from landfills.

### 6. Learn About Labels:
Familiarize yourself with food labels like "organic," "fair trade," and "cage-free." These labels can indicate more sustainable and ethical production methods.

### 7. Choose Ethical Meat and Dairy:
If you consume animal products, seek out meat and dairy from sources that prioritize animal welfare and use sustainable farming practices.

### 8. Support Local Farmers' Markets:
Shop at farmers' markets to connect with local growers and access fresh, seasonal produce.

### 9. Reduce Single-Use Plastic:
Cut down on single-use plastic by using reusable shopping bags, containers, and water bottles. Avoid products with excessive packaging.

### 10. Educate Yourself:
- Stay informed about food production, agricultural practices, and sustainability. Understanding the food system empowers you to make informed choices.

### 11. Conserve Water:
Consider the water footprint of your food choices. Some foods, like meat, require a significant amount of water to produce. Being mindful of this can help conserve this vital resource.

### 12. Support Food Access Initiatives:
Contribute to food access programs and initiatives in your community to help combat food insecurity.

### 13. Reduce Fast Food and Highly Processed Foods:
Fast food and highly processed foods often have negative social and environmental consequences. Reducing your consumption of these items can lead to healthier and more sustainable eating.

### 14. Grow Your Own:
If possible, start a garden or grow herbs and vegetables at home. This promotes a closer connection to your food and reduces the need for transportation.

### *15. Advocate for Change:*

*Use your voice to advocate for sustainable and ethical food policies and practices in your local community and beyond.*

*By making sustainable and ethical food choices, you can contribute to a healthier planet, support fair and humane treatment of animals, and promote the well-being of communities. These choices not only benefit you but also have far-reaching positive impacts on the environment and society as a whole.*

# CHAPTER 42

## Food and Mood: The Gut-Brain Connection

*The relationship between what we eat and how we feel is a fascinating area of research known as the gut-brain connection. It explores how the food we consume can influence our mood, mental health, and overall well-being. Here's an overview of this complex relationship:*

### 1. Gut Microbiota:

*The gut is home to trillions of microorganisms, collectively known as the gut microbiota. These microorganisms play a crucial role in digestion and also impact brain health.*

### 2. The Vagus Nerve:

*The gut is connected to the brain through the vagus nerve, which allows bidirectional communication. Signals travel from the gut to the brain and vice versa.*

### 3. Neurotransmitters:

*The gut produces many of the same neurotransmitters as the brain, including serotonin, which is often referred to as the "feel-good" hormone. An estimated 90% of serotonin is produced in the gut.*

### 4. Inflammation:
*An imbalanced gut microbiota can lead to chronic inflammation, which has been linked to mood disorders like depression and anxiety.*

### 5. Nutrient Intake:
*The food we eat provides essential nutrients that support brain function. Nutrient deficiencies can affect mood and cognitive health.*

### 6. Probiotics and Prebiotics:
*Consuming foods rich in probiotics (good bacteria) and prebiotics (food for good bacteria) can help maintain a healthy gut microbiota and potentially improve mood.*

### 7. Connection to Mental Health:
*Emerging research suggests that an imbalanced gut microbiota may contribute to mental health conditions, including depression, anxiety, and even conditions like autism and schizophrenia.*

### 8. Diet and Mental Health:
*A diet high in processed foods, sugars, and unhealthy fats may contribute to poor mental health, while a diet rich in whole foods, fiber, and healthy fats can have a positive impact.*

### 9. Individual Variability:

*The gut-brain connection is complex, and its effects can vary among individuals. What works for one person may not work the same way for another.*

### 10. Lifestyle Factors:
*Factors like stress, sleep, and physical activity can also influence the gut-brain connection. Reducing stress and getting adequate sleep are crucial for maintaining a healthy gut and promoting good mental health.*

### 11. Personalized Nutrition:
*Some researchers are exploring the concept of "personalized nutrition" to tailor dietary recommendations based on an individual's unique gut microbiota and health goals.*

### 12. Clinical Applications:
*The gut-brain connection is an area of active research, and while it holds promise for mental health interventions, it is not a substitute for professional treatment for conditions like depression and anxiety.*

*Understanding the gut-brain connection highlights the importance of a balanced diet, rich in fruits, vegetables, whole grains, lean proteins, and healthy fats, for both physical and mental health. While food can influence mood, it's just one piece of the complex puzzle that is mental well-being.*

# CHAPTER 43

## Nutrition and Exercise: A Dynamic Duo for Health

*Nutrition and exercise are two pillars of a healthy lifestyle. When combined effectively, they have a synergistic impact on your overall well-being. Here's how they complement each other:*

### 1. Energy Balance:
*Nutrition provides the energy (calories) your body needs to fuel physical activity. Balancing calorie intake with expenditure is essential for maintaining a healthy weight.*

### 2. Performance and Recovery:
*Proper nutrition supports physical performance and aids in post-exercise recovery. Carbohydrates provide energy, protein repairs and builds muscles, and fats fuel endurance activities.*

### 3. Muscle Health:
*Adequate protein intake is crucial for building and maintaining lean muscle mass. Amino acids from protein sources are the building blocks of muscle tissue.*

### *4. Hydration:*
*Staying well-hydrated is vital for exercise performance and overall health. Water is necessary for various bodily functions, including temperature regulation.*

### **5. Macronutrients and Micronutrients:**
*Carbohydrates, fats, and protein are macronutrients that provide energy. Micronutrients like vitamins and minerals support metabolic processes, bone health, and immunity.*

### **6. Timing Matters:**
*When you eat can impact your workouts. Eating a balanced meal or snack before exercise provides energy, while a post-workout meal supports recovery.*

### **7. Weight Management:**
*Combining a healthy diet with regular physical activity is effective for weight management. Exercise burns calories, and proper nutrition helps control calorie intake.*

### **8. Cardiovascular Health:**
*Regular exercise and a heart-healthy diet can improve cardiovascular health by reducing the risk of heart disease, lowering blood pressure, and improving cholesterol levels.*

### **9. Bone Health:**

Adequate calcium and vitamin D intake, along with weight-bearing exercise, supports strong bones and reduces the risk of osteoporosis.

### 10. Mental Health:
Exercise releases endorphins, which can improve mood and reduce stress. A balanced diet with essential nutrients supports brain function and mental well-being.

### 11. Long-Term Health Benefits:
Regular physical activity and a healthy diet contribute to a lower risk of chronic diseases such as type 2 diabetes, certain cancers, and hypertension.

### 12. Weight Loss:
While exercise aids in burning calories, weight loss primarily depends on creating a calorie deficit through a combination of diet and physical activity.

### 13. Individual Needs:
Everyone's nutritional and exercise needs are different. Factors like age, gender, activity level, and health conditions play a role in determining the best approach for each person.

### 14. Professional Guidance:
Consultation with a registered dietitian and or a fitness professional can help tailor your nutrition and exercise plan to your unique goals and needs.

*Nutrition and exercise are integral components of a healthy lifestyle. Together, they can enhance your quality of life, improve your physical and mental well-being, and help you achieve your health and fitness goals. It's important to strike a balance that suits your individual needs and preferences.*

# CHAPTER 44

## Weight Management Strategies: Achieving and Maintaining a Healthy Weight

*Maintaining a healthy weight is essential for overall well-being and can reduce the risk of many health conditions. Here are some effective weight management strategies to help you achieve and maintain a healthy weight:*

### 1. Balanced Diet:

*Consume a balanced diet rich in fruits, vegetables, whole grains, lean proteins, and healthy fats. Avoid or limit foods high in added sugars, saturated fats, and processed ingredients.*

### 2. Portion Control:

*Be mindful of portion sizes to avoid overeating. Use smaller plates, bowls, and utensils to help control portion sizes.*

### 3. Regular Meals:

*Eat regular meals and snacks to maintain steady energy levels and prevent excessive hunger, which can lead to overeating.*

### 4. Mindful Eating:
Pay attention to what you eat, savor your food, and eat without distractions. This can help you recognize when you're full and prevent overconsumption.

### 5. Hydration:
Stay well-hydrated by drinking water throughout the day. Sometimes, thirst can be mistaken for hunger.

### 6. Limit Processed Foods:
Processed foods are often high in calories, sugar, and unhealthy fats. Minimize your intake of these items.

### 7. Regular Exercise:
Incorporate regular physical activity into your routine. A combination of cardiovascular exercise, strength training, and flexibility exercises can help you burn calories and maintain muscle mass.

### 8. Set Realistic Goals:
Set achievable, realistic weight loss or maintenance goals. Small, sustainable changes are more effective than drastic ones.

### 9. Track Your Progress:
Keep a food diary or use a tracking app to monitor your eating habits and physical activity. This can help you identify areas for improvement.

### 10. Seek Professional Guidance:

*Consider consulting with a registered dietitian or a fitness professional who can provide personalized guidance and support.*

### 11. Emotional Eating Awareness:
*Be mindful of emotional eating. Learn to recognize your emotional triggers and find alternative ways to cope with stress, sadness, or boredom.*

### 12. Sleep:
*Prioritize quality sleep. Lack of sleep can disrupt hormones that regulate appetite and lead to weight gain.*

### 13. Meal Planning and Prepping:
*Plan your meals and snacks in advance to avoid impulsive, unhealthy choices. Prepping healthy options can help you stay on track.*

### 14. Support System:
*Engage with a supportive network of friends, family, or a weight management group. Accountability and encouragement can be valuable.*

### 15. Slow, Sustainable Changes:
*Avoid fad diets or extreme weight loss methods. Slow and steady changes are more likely to lead to long-term success.*

### 16. Focus on Health, Not Just Appearance:

*Prioritize your health and well-being over appearance-based goals. This mindset can lead to more sustainable choices.*

### 17. Stay Positive:
*Maintain a positive attitude and practice self-compassion. Weight management is a journey, and setbacks are a normal part of the process.*

### 18. Weight Maintenance:
*Remember that maintaining a healthy weight is just as important as losing weight. Focus on long-term health and well-being.*

*Effective weight management involves a combination of healthy eating, regular physical activity, and a supportive lifestyle. It's not just about losing weight; it's about making sustainable choices that promote lifelong health and well-being.*

# CHAPTER 45

## Diabetes and Nutrition: Managing Blood Sugar Through Diet

*For individuals with diabetes, proper nutrition plays a pivotal role in managing blood sugar levels and overall health. Whether you have type 1, type 2, or gestational diabetes, here's how nutrition can help:*

### 1. Carbohydrate Management:

*Carbohydrates have the most significant impact on blood sugar levels. Monitor your carbohydrate intake and spread it evenly throughout the day. Choose complex carbohydrates like whole grains, fruits, and vegetables over simple sugars.*

### 2. Portion Control:

*Pay attention to portion sizes to prevent overeating, which can cause blood sugar spikes. Measuring and weighing food can be helpful.*

### 3. Glycemic Index:

*Consider the glycemic index (GI) of foods. Low-GI foods have a milder impact on blood sugar levels* compared to high-GI foods. Focus on low-GI options like quinoa, legumes, and non-starchy vegetables.

### 4. Balanced Meals:
Create balanced meals that include lean protein sources, healthy fats, and fiber-rich carbohydrates. This combination helps stabilize blood sugar levels and keeps you satisfied.

### 5. Fiber:
Foods high in fiber, such as whole grains, beans, and vegetables, can slow the absorption of sugar and improve blood sugar control.

### 6. Sugar and Sweeteners:
Limit your intake of added sugars and artificial sweeteners. Opt for natural sweeteners like stevia or small amounts of honey or maple syrup, if needed.

### 7. Regular Meals:
Stick to regular meal times and avoid skipping meals. Consistency in your eating schedule helps regulate blood sugar.

### 8. Monitoring Blood Sugar:
Keep track of your blood sugar levels as directed by your healthcare provider. This information can guide your dietary choices and insulin or medication management.

### 9. Hydration:

Stay well-hydrated, as dehydration can affect blood sugar levels. Drink water, herbal teas, or other low-calorie beverages.

### 10. Healthy Fats:
Include sources of healthy fats, such as avocados, nuts, seeds, and olive oil, in your diet. These fats help with satiety and support overall health.

### 11. Limit Processed Foods:
Processed foods often contain hidden sugars and unhealthy fats. Minimize your consumption of these items.

### 12. Meal Planning
Plan your meals and snacks in advance to maintain better control over your food choices.

### 13. Individualized Care:
Diabetes management is highly individualized. Work closely with your healthcare team, including a registered dietitian, to create a meal plan that suits your specific needs and preferences.

### 14. Regular Exercise:
Combine proper nutrition with regular physical activity to further improve blood sugar control and overall health.

### 15. Medication and Insulin:

*If you're on medication or insulin, coordinate your meal plan with your medication schedule to avoid blood sugar fluctuations.*

### 16. Blood Pressure and Cholesterol:
*Manage other risk factors like high blood pressure and high cholesterol, as these are often associated with diabetes.*

*Effective diabetes management through nutrition requires a combination of education, self-awareness, and consistent choices. By making informed food decisions, monitoring your blood sugar levels, and working closely with your healthcare team, you can improve your blood sugar control and overall quality of life.*

# CHAPTER 46

## Heart Health and Nutrition: A Guide to Cardiovascular Well-Being

*Maintaining heart health through proper nutrition is crucial in preventing heart disease and supporting overall well-being. Here's a guide to how nutrition can positively impact your cardiovascular health:*

### 1. Heart-Healthy Diet:
*Consume a heart-healthy diet that focuses on nutrient-rich, whole foods. This includes plenty of fruits, vegetables, whole grains, lean proteins, and healthy fats like those found in nuts, seeds, and olive oil.*

### 2. Limit Saturated and Trans Fats:
*Reduce your intake of saturated and trans fats, often found in red meat, processed foods, and fried items. These fats can raise bad cholesterol levels (LDL).*

### 3. Choose Unsaturated Fats:
*Opt for unsaturated fats like those in avocados, fatty fish, and nuts. These fats can help lower bad cholesterol and improve heart health.*

### 4. Fiber Intake:

*Increase your fiber intake from sources like whole grains, legumes, and vegetables. Fiber helps lower cholesterol levels and supports heart health.*

### 5. Omega-3 Fatty Acids:

*Incorporate sources of omega-3 fatty acids, such as salmon, flaxseeds, and walnuts, into your diet. Omega-3s can reduce the risk of heart disease.*

### 6. Sodium Reduction:

*Lower your sodium intake by limiting processed and restaurant foods. Excessive sodium can contribute to high blood pressure, a risk factor for heart disease.*

### 7. Control Portion Sizes:

*Be mindful of portion sizes to avoid overeating, which can lead to weight gain and increased risk of heart disease.*

### 8. Limit Added Sugars:

*Minimize your consumption of added sugars found in sugary beverages and processed foods. High sugar intake can contribute to obesity and heart disease.*

### 9. Hydration:

*Stay well-hydrated with water, as dehydration can affect blood pressure and overall heart health.*

### 10. Meal Planning:

*Plan your meals and snacks to ensure you have access to heart-healthy options throughout the day.*

### 11. Nutrient Balance:

*Strive for balanced meals that include a variety of nutrients. A balanced diet supports overall health and can help with weight management.*

### 12. Alcohol Moderation:

*If you consume alcohol, do so in moderation. Excessive alcohol can lead to high blood pressure and other heart-related issues.*

### 13. Regular Exercise:

*Combine proper nutrition with regular physical activity to improve cardiovascular health, manage weight, and reduce the risk of heart disease.*

### 14. Regular Health Screenings:

*Schedule regular health check-ups to monitor your heart health, blood pressure, cholesterol levels, and other risk factors.*

### 15. Smoking Cessation:

*If you smoke, consider quitting. Smoking is a major risk factor for heart disease.*

### 16. Stress Management:

*Practice stress-reduction techniques like mindfulness, meditation, and deep breathing to protect your heart from the negative effects of chronic stress.*

### *17. Personalized Approach:*

*Heart health is individual. Consider consulting with a healthcare provider or registered dietitian for personalized guidance.*

*A heart-healthy diet combined with other lifestyle factors, like regular exercise and stress management, can significantly reduce your risk of heart disease. Remember that small, sustainable changes in your eating habits and lifestyle can have a profound impact on your cardiovascular well-being.*

# CHAPTER 47

## Nutrition for Bone Health: Building and Maintaining Strong Bones:

*Proper nutrition is essential for building and maintaining strong, healthy bones. Whether you're aiming to support bone development in your youth or maintain bone density as you age, here's how nutrition can help:*

### 1. Calcium:
*Calcium is a fundamental mineral for bone health. Include dairy products, leafy green vegetables, fortified plant-based milk, and fortified foods in your diet to meet your calcium needs.*

### 2. Vitamin D:
*Vitamin D is crucial for calcium absorption. Get adequate sun exposure and consume vitamin D-rich foods like fatty fish (salmon, mackerel), egg yolks, and fortified products.*

### 3. Vitamin K:

Vitamin K plays a role in bone mineralization. Leafy greens (kale, spinach), broccoli, and Brussels sprouts are excellent sources.

### 4. Magnesium:
Magnesium is necessary for calcium absorption and bone health. Include magnesium-rich foods like nuts, seeds, whole grains, and dark chocolate in your diet.

### 5. Phosphorus:
Phosphorus is another mineral essential for bone health. It's abundant in foods like meat, poultry, fish, dairy products, and nuts.

### 6. Protein:
Protein provides amino acids needed for bone growth and repair. Include lean protein sources like poultry, fish, legumes, and dairy in your diet.

### 7. Collagen:
Collagen is a protein that contributes to bone strength and flexibility. You can find it in bone broth, chicken skin, and supplements.

### 8. Omega-3 Fatty Acids:
Omega-3s from fatty fish (salmon, sardines) and flaxseeds may reduce the risk of osteoporosis and support bone health.

### 9. Limit Salt Intake:

*High sodium intake can lead to calcium loss from bones. Reduce your consumption of processed and salty foods.*

### 10. Alkaline Diet:

*Some evidence suggests that an alkaline diet, which focuses on fruits and vegetables, may support bone health by reducing calcium loss.*

### 11. Limit Caffeine and Alcohol:

*Excessive caffeine and alcohol can interfere with calcium absorption. Moderate your intake of these beverages.*

### 12. Weight-Bearing Exercise:

*Combine proper nutrition with weight-bearing exercises like walking, running, or weightlifting to strengthen bones.*

### 13. Avoid Smoking:

*Smoking has been linked to bone loss. Quitting smoking can benefit your overall bone health.*

### 14. Maintain a Healthy Weight:

*Maintaining a healthy weight is important for bone health. Extreme underweight or obesity can both lead to bone issues.*

### 15. Hormonal Health:

*Ensure hormonal balance, especially for women during menopause, as hormonal changes can affect bone density.*

### 16. Regular Health Check-Ups:
*Schedule regular check-ups to monitor your bone health, especially if you have risk factors or a family history of bone-related conditions.*

*A well-balanced diet that includes these nutrients, combined with a healthy lifestyle, can contribute to strong and resilient bones. It's never too early or too late to prioritize bone health through proper nutrition and other preventive measures.*

# CHAPTER 48

## Nutrition and Cancer Prevention: A Dietary Approach to Reduce Risk

*While there are no guarantees when it comes to preventing cancer, certain dietary choices and habits can reduce your risk. Here's how nutrition plays a vital role in cancer prevention:*

### 1. Eat a Variety of Fruits and Vegetables:
*These foods are rich in vitamins, minerals, and antioxidants that help protect against cell damage and reduce the risk of several types of cancer. Aim for a colorful mix of produce.*

### 2. High-Fiber Diet:
*Foods high in fiber, such as whole grains, legumes, and vegetables, can help reduce the risk of colorectal cancer. Fiber aids in digestion and may help remove potentially harmful substances from the body.*

### 3. Lean Protein Sources:

*Choose lean protein sources like poultry, fish, and plant-based proteins over red and processed meats. High consumption of red and processed meats is associated with an increased risk of cancer, particularly colorectal cancer.*

### 4. Healthy Fats:
*Opt for healthy fats from sources like avocados, nuts, seeds, and olive oil. Reducing saturated and trans fats can lower the risk of various cancers.*

### 5. Limit Added Sugars:
*High sugar intake may contribute to obesity and chronic inflammation, both of which are risk factors for cancer. Minimize sugary beverages and processed sweets.*

### 6. Antioxidants:
*Antioxidant-rich foods, such as berries, citrus fruits, and green tea, help protect cells from damage. Antioxidants can potentially reduce the risk of cancer.*

### 7. Hydration:
*Staying well-hydrated is essential. Water helps with digestion and the elimination of waste products from the body.*

### 8. Portion Control:
*Maintain a healthy weight through portion control. Being overweight or obese is linked to a higher risk of certain cancers.*

### 9. Alcohol Moderation:

*Limit alcohol consumption. Excessive alcohol intake is associated with an increased risk of several types of cancer.*

### 10. Phytochemicals:

*Include foods rich in phytochemicals, like cruciferous vegetables (broccoli, cauliflower) and garlic, in your diet. These substances may help protect against cancer.*

### 11. Cooking Methods:

*Choose healthier cooking methods like grilling, steaming, and baking. Avoid charring or overcooking meat, as this can produce carcinogenic substances.*

### 12. Avoid Processed Foods:

*Highly processed and ultra-processed foods often contain additives and preservatives that may have carcinogenic potential. Focus on whole, unprocessed foods.*

### 13. Food Quality:

*Prioritize food quality over quantity. Eating nutrient-dense, whole foods provides essential nutrients and minimizes exposure to potentially harmful substances.*

### 14. Consult a Registered Dietitian:

*If you have specific dietary concerns or are at higher risk for cancer due to family history or other factors, consider seeking guidance from a registered dietitian.*

*Remember that cancer risk is influenced by a combination of factors, including genetics, environment, and lifestyle. While nutrition plays a significant role, maintaining a healthy lifestyle that includes regular exercise, not smoking, and protecting your skin from excessive sun exposure are also essential in cancer prevention. Always consult with a healthcare professional for personalized guidance and early cancer screenings.*

# CHAPTER 49

## Nutritional Considerations for Chronic Diseases: Managing Health Through Diet

*Diet plays a crucial role in the management and prevention of chronic diseases. Here are some nutritional considerations for common chronic conditions:*

### 1. Heart Disease:
*Focus on a heart-healthy diet that's low in saturated fats, trans fats, and sodium. Include fruits, vegetables, whole grains, lean proteins, and healthy fats. Omega-3 fatty acids from fatty fish can help reduce the risk of heart disease.*

### 2. Diabetes:
*Monitor carbohydrate intake to control blood sugar levels. Choose complex carbohydrates, high-fiber foods, and lean proteins. Consistency in meal timing and portion control is important for diabetes management.*

### 3. Hypertension (High Blood Pressure):

*Reduce sodium intake, eat potassium-rich foods like bananas and leafy greens, and maintain a healthy weight. The DASH (Dietary Approaches to Stop Hypertension) diet is a good guideline.*

### 4. Obesity:
*Focus on a well-balanced, calorie-controlled diet to achieve and maintain a healthy weight. Portion control, mindful eating, and regular physical activity are key.*

### 5. Osteoporosis:
*Ensure adequate calcium and vitamin D intake. Include dairy products, fortified plant-based milk, leafy greens, and weight-bearing exercises for bone health.*

### 6. Kidney Disease:
*Adjust protein, sodium, and phosphorus intake based on the stage of kidney disease. Work with a registered dietitian to develop a personalized plan.*

### 7. Gastrointestinal Disorders (e.g., IBS, Crohn's Disease):
*Identify trigger foods and manage symptoms with a low-FODMAP diet or other recommended dietary changes. Fiber and probiotics may also be beneficial.*

### 8. Cancer:
*Focus on an anti-inflammatory diet rich in fruits, vegetables, and antioxidants. Limit processed meats and sugary foods. Adequate protein intake is essential for muscle maintenance during treatment.*

### 9. Respiratory Conditions (e.g., Asthma):

Consume foods high in antioxidants and anti-inflammatory compounds, such as fruits, vegetables, and omega-3 fatty acids from fish.

### 10. Alzheimer's Disease and Cognitive Decline:

A Mediterranean-style diet, rich in fruits, vegetables, whole grains, and healthy fats, has been associated with cognitive health. Antioxidants and omega-3 fatty acids may be protective.

### 11. Autoimmune Diseases:

Dietary approaches can vary for different autoimmune diseases. In some cases, an anti-inflammatory diet, such as the Mediterranean diet, can be beneficial. Others may require specific dietary modifications.

### 12. Gout:

Limit high-purine foods like red meat and organ meats. Maintain a healthy weight and stay well-hydrated to reduce the risk of gout attacks.

### 13. Celiac Disease:

Completely eliminate gluten-containing grains like wheat, barley, and rye from your diet. Focus on gluten-free grains, fruits, vegetables, and lean proteins.

### 14. Food Allergies:

*Avoid allergenic foods and carefully read food labels to prevent exposure to allergens. Work with a healthcare provider or dietitian for guidance.*

### 15. Mental Health Conditions:
*Diet can influence mental health. Include whole foods, omega-3 fatty acids, and probiotics in your diet. Limit processed and sugary foods.*

*For any chronic disease, it's essential to work closely with healthcare providers and registered dietitians to develop a personalized nutrition plan. Remember that diet is just one aspect of managing chronic conditions, and it should be integrated with other treatment strategies and a healthy lifestyle.*

# CHAPTER 50

## The Future of Nutrition: Trends and Innovations

*The field of nutrition is continuously evolving, and several trends and innovations are shaping its future. Here's a glimpse into what we can expect:*

### 1. Personalized Nutrition:
*Advances in genetics and technology are enabling tailored dietary recommendations based on an individual's unique genetic makeup, metabolism, and health goals.*

### 2. Functional Foods:
*Functional foods are designed to offer specific health benefits beyond basic nutrition. We can expect an increasing variety of foods fortified with probiotics, prebiotics, antioxidants, and other bioactive compounds.*

### 3. Plant-Based Eating:
*Plant-based diets are on the rise due to environmental, health, and ethical concerns. More plant-based alternatives to meat and dairy products are emerging, catering to a growing demand.*

### 4. Sustainable Nutrition:

Sustainability is becoming a central focus. People are more conscious of the environmental impact of their food choices, leading to trends like reduced food waste and farm-to-table eating.

### 5. Nutrigenomics

The study of how nutrients interact with an individual's genes is expanding. Nutrigenomics may offer insights into how dietary choices can affect disease risk and management.

### 6. AI and Nutrition Apps:

Artificial intelligence and nutrition apps are making it easier to track dietary intake, receive personalized meal plans, and access nutrition-related information.

### 7. Gut Health:

A deeper understanding of the gut microbiome's impact on overall health is leading to dietary recommendations that focus on improving gut health through prebiotics, probiotics, and fiber-rich foods.

### 8. Insect-Based Protein:

Insects are being explored as a sustainable and protein-rich food source. Insect-based protein products are gaining attention for their nutritional and environmental benefits.

### 9. Precision Nutrition:

*Precision nutrition takes a holistic approach to health by considering factors like genetics, lifestyle, and environment when creating personalized dietary plans.*

### 10. Lab-Grown Meat:
*The development of lab-grown meat and cell-cultured proteins aims to reduce the environmental impact of traditional meat production.*

### 11. Nutritional Supplements:
*Innovative supplements, such as personalized vitamins and minerals based on individual needs, are expected to gain popularity.*

### 12. Food as Medicine:
*More focus is shifting toward using food as a preventative and therapeutic tool for managing chronic diseases and conditions.*

### 13. Allergen-Free Foods:
*Increasing awareness of food allergies and intolerances is driving the development of a wider range of allergen-free products.*

### 14. Food Transparency:
*Consumers are demanding more transparency in the food industry, pushing for clearer labeling, traceability, and access to information about the sources and production processes of their food.*

### 15. Virtual Nutrition Counseling:

*Telehealth and virtual consultations with registered dietitians are becoming more common, making nutrition guidance more accessible.*

*As technology, science, and consumer preferences continue to evolve, the future of nutrition will likely be marked by greater personalization, sustainability, and a deeper understanding of the intricate relationship between diet and health. Staying informed and adapting to these trends can help individuals make more informed and healthier dietary choices.*

# CHAPTER 51

## Conclusion: The Power of Nutrition and Diet in Our Lives

***Nutrition and diet*** *are not just about the foods we consume; they are about the fundamental building blocks of our health and well-being. The impact of our dietary choices extends far beyond satisfying hunger – it shapes our longevity, our resistance to disease, and the quality of our lives.*

*In this journey through **nutrition and diet,** we have explored the critical role of macronutrients and micronutrients, dissected the anatomy of our digestive system, and delved into the intricacies of special diets. We've learned about the significance of nutrition at different life stages and the vital link between food and mood.a*

*We've seen that proper nutrition is not a one-size-fits-all concept; it's highly individual and adaptable to our unique needs and goals. Nutrition can prevent and manage chronic diseases, fuel our physical activities, and support healthy aging. It can even be a form of medicine, as the saying goes, "Let food be thy medicine and medicine be thy food."*

*The future of nutrition holds exciting possibilities with personalized diets, functional foods, and innovations that cater to our ever-evolving health and environmental concerns. As we stand at the crossroads of a new era in nutrition, the choices we make about what we eat will shape not only our own health but also the health of the planet.*

*Ultimately, **nutrition and diet** are a lifelong journey. They are about making informed choices and cultivating healthy habits. It's about finding balance, seeking variety, and respecting the profound connection between what we consume and how we live.*

*So, as we navigate the vast landscape of nutrition, let's remember that the power to transform our lives through diet lies within our reach. With knowledge, mindfulness, and a commitment to our well-being, we can savor the benefits of a healthy, nutritious, and fulfilling life.*